CHAIR YOGA FOR SENIORS

Quick and Easy Low Impact Exercises for Weight Loss, Improved Mobility, and Independence in Under 10 Minutes a Day

MARGARET BRUNNER

Copyright © 2023
MARGARET BRUNNER
CHAIR YOGA FOR SENIORS
Quick and Easy Low Impact Exercises for Weight Loss, Improved Mobility, and Independence in Under 10 Minutes a Day
All rights reserved.

No part of this publication may be reproduced, distributed, or transmitted in any form or by any means, including photocopying, recording, or other electronic or mechanical methods, without the prior written permission of the author, except in the case of brief quotations embodied in critical reviews and certain other non-commercial uses permitted by copyright law.

MARGARET BRUNNER

Printed Worldwide
First Printing 2023
First Edition 2023

10 9 8 7 6 5 4 3 2 1

CHAIR YOGA FOR SENIORS

Table of Contents

CHAIR YOGA 1
   INTRODUCTION 2
   CHAPTER ONE 6
      SENIOR FITNESS 6
   CHAPTER TWO 16
      THE CONCEPT OF CHAIR YOGA 16
   CHAPTER THREE 21
      CHAIR YOGA POSTURES 21
   CHAPTER FOUR 46
      MORE CHAIR YOGA POSTURES 46
   CONCLUSION 61

BALANCE & FALL PREVENTION PROGRAM 62
   INTRODUCTION 63
   CHAPTER ONE 69
      BONE HEALTH & BALANCE 69
   CHAPTER TWO 76
      METHODS TO IMPROVE BALANCE AND BODY STRENGTH 76
   CHAPTER THREE 84
      EXERCISES TO IMPROVE BALANCE & PREVENT FALLS 84
   CHAPTER FOUR 89
      ASANAS TO IMPROVE STRENGTH 89
   CHAPTER FIVE 103
      SOME MORE ASANAS 103
   CONCLUSION 112

MINDFUL CHAIR YOGA 113
   INTRODUCTION 114
   CHAPTER ONE 120
      MENTAL HEALTH IN WOMEN 120
   CHAPTER TWO 127
      STRESS AND MANAGEMENT OF STRESS IN WOMEN OF AGE GROUP FIFTY TO SEVENTY AND ABOVE 127
   CHAPTER THREE 134
      POSITIVE PSYCHOLOGY, MINDFULNESS, AND YOGA 134
   CHAPTER FOUR 140
      ASANAS TO REDUCE STRESS 140
   CHAPTER FIVE 158

- *Breathing And Mindful Yoga* *158*
- CONCLUSION 166
- **STRONG BONES FOR SENIORS** **167**
- INTRODUCTION 168
- CHAPTER ONE 173
  - *What Is Osteoporosis?* *173*
- CHAPTER TWO 179
  - *Osteoporosis Diagnosis* *179*
- CHAPTER THREE 185
  - *Osteoporosis Management & Prevention* *185*
- CHAPTER FOUR 193
  - *Weight-Bearing Chair Yoga Exercises* *193*
- CHAPTER FIVE 214
  - *Gentle Yoga for Osteoporosis* *214*
- CONCLUSION 229

BONUS

Receive your FREE AUDIO BOOK of Margaret Brunner's "Chair Yoga for Seniors" and listen to step-by-step directions of the exercises in the comfort of your home or when you're out and about, without carrying a physical book.

To claim your FREE AUDIO BOOK and gain access to a number of other bonuses to support you on your journey to fitness and and maintaining a healthy lifestyle go to link:

https://rb.gy/s2py6

Chair Yoga

Fully Illustrated Exercise Routines to Comfortably Reduce Joint Pain and Increase Joint Flexibility with only 10 minutes a Day.

Introduction

"Aging is not lost youth but a new stage of opportunity and strength."
-Betty Friedan

Let's look at a picture together. This one, on the bookshelf, is just right. It is so optimistic, bright, and cheerful. It is of you with your son and husband. You are looking up at them, your eyes sparkling, and your face lit up in a glorious smile— for it is the glory of youth, a force formidable—your skin glistens. Your eyes have a twinkle in them, amplifying the carefree exuberance with which you grin. Those were the times when the hair was naturally black, the skin was taut, and the body was deft and flexible. Much like youth, they are all gone with the blowing wind.

That picture is from when you were darting, dashing, and racing through life. You were busy with your chores, raising two children, and managing your home and work. You flitted from task to task, each no less important than the other. Thoughts about old age and creaking joints or a ramrod body refusing to comply per necessity were abstract. And this is natural because the concept of fifty seems strangely remote and detached at twenty-five.

In your list of priorities, you had no allocations for exercise or disciplined self-care routines; there simply wasn't enough time. It was essential to run errands, prepare family meals, clean the house, accompany your son to school or Karate classes, and fetch him. You had your job to worry about. Your days started early and ended late. You were there for everyone, for they were all your responsibility.

Regarding exercise, you thought you were getting enough of it. Weren't you up and running all the time? Truth be told, you felt so tired that as soon as your head touched the pillow at night, you were off to sleep.

Consequently, you did no other fitness activity besides your routine work.

Time passed, and life became sedentary. You found that age made it difficult for you to be as active as you once were. You always thought you were super-active! So, what went wrong?

Aging itself can cause joint and muscle stiffness and pain, coupled with a sedentary lifestyle and time spent indoors. Obesity, smoking, or excessive drinking are associated with bone and joint problems. Osteoarthritis, muscle weakness, or sensory affection can debilitate many others. Mental illnesses, like depression, can prevent exercise, causing bone and muscle wasting.

How considering movement difficulties as *challenges* might help us?

A challenge mindset recognises that changes will undoubtedly occur per natural law. When we accept it for what it is, we acknowledge that our bodies and mind change over time. While our bodies get less pliable, aging increases the level of wisdom we accrued in life.

Manipulating certainties with wishful thinking never helps; contrarily, it diminishes our courage and fortitude. A challenging mindset can enable us to accept and handle situations honestly and clearly.

We analyze adversity to understand what we can do about it without succumbing to it. While we may not have anything to lose, we may gain a lot.

We analyze three things:

- How the situation or the condition affects us, and whether we care about it.

- Assessing whether we have the resources to address the situation. If we surrender, thinking, we do not have the means to face the situation, it becomes a threat. Challenging ourselves to face the problem with an open mind is more optimistic.
- We gain the lessons learned to form new experiences throughout the process. It is to bolster the growth mentality to prevent mental aging.

Challenge mindset leads to emotional resilience, the first crucial step toward gaining overall health.

Our challenge is to be able to do our grocery shopping again. We want to prepare our meals, tidy up our rooms, and fold our clothes— the marvellous mundane that has become tough.

What resources can we explore to improve mobility and reduce body pain and aches? Multiple well-documented studies have shown that daily yoga for as little as ten minutes can favor our physical and mental well-being. It delays cellular aging and prevents the decline of cognitive functions, among other benefits.

Yoga also helps maintain joint mobility and joint sense, called proprioception. They are essential for posture and balance. Consequently, the chances of falls are reduced.

Anyone can participate in yoga practice. It can be *modified* for all ages and groups.

Yoga is Sanskrit for *yog*, meaning to add or *union*. The discipline includes physical, mental, and spiritual practices to regulate our minds and bodies. It works on the precept that we can control only one thing: ourselves. We must aim to understand our sentiments, wishes, and potential and take responsibility.

It is within our power to achieve happiness and contentment in life. To do so, we must be aware of our thoughts, beliefs, and feelings, probe them, and reflect if modifying them will make us happier and more fulfilled. We possess the key to happiness when we function from a "we can" mentality.

In my long career as a yoga instructor, I have been honored to work alongside many yoga gurus. While working with my senior students, I discovered their emotional strength in overcoming physical constraints. They had independently handled their adult lives and were not prepared to settle for any less in their old age.

Their passion and grit impressed me, and I researched which aspects of yoga could help them more. I also studied and analyzed methods to create a strategy that would be helpful for seniors with mobility issues, like standing for a considerable time or flexing body parts to the full extent.

I found chair yoga a valuable option for practicing different postures and movements. It improved body and mind agility and eventually reduced joint stiffness and pain. Seniors above 65 can easily participate in this inclusive practice and gain the same benefits as standard yoga training.

I compiled the especially beneficial poses for improving flexibility and reducing muscle and joint stiffness and pain. Use these simple-to-do curated exercises to enjoy little moments of self-satisfaction. You feel happy doing them and love what you can do independently.

My book serves to guide you through this journey of self-discovery. The first chapter of the book discusses fitness for seniors and age-related issues. Chapter two is on how chair yoga can help you. Chapters three and four are on different postures, cool-down, and warm-up techniques.

Let's delve into the treasure of health and fitness without delay.

Chapter One

Senior Fitness

"Age is a matter of feeling, not of years."

-George William Curtis

The concept of fitness as a means to adapt to the environment is embedded in the history of human evolution. "The fittest survived" was the *mantra*, not only of the jungle world but also of our civilization. The current definition of fitness also involves mental and emotional well-being.

History of Fitness

Ancient Egyptians and ancient Chinese were said to have structured acrobatics programs. Ancient Europe learned fitness from the Greeks, who designed formal athletic training. Plato noted that lack of activity deteriorated health, but mobility and exercise preserved it. He emphasized the exercise must be systematized and not just any training.

Post-industrialized world, particularly after World War II, embraced the term fitness and applied it to the ability to perform and adapt to varying conditions. It includes *muscle strength* and *endurance*, *cardiorespiratory endurance*, *balance*, *flexibility*, and *speed*. *Body composition* measurement in fitness assesses the visceral fat surrounding vital organs like the heart, liver, and kidney. As opposed to subcutaneous fat, which protects us from cold and exposure, visceral fat indicates basal metabolic rate (BMI), a benchmark of appropriate weight for the height of an individual.

Definition

The Centers for Disease Control and Prevention (CDC) defines physical fitness as the ability to do our daily tasks with energy and agility. We must be vigorous enough to respond to emergencies. We are not fatigued by our activities and have enough enthusiasm to pursue leisure activities.

CDC believes regular physical activity is one of the most vital preventative methods to stop or check several illnesses, including chronic lifestyle illnesses like type 2 diabetes mellitus and hypertension. Older adults risk degenerative diseases most because of the natural inclination to slow down and become more sedentary.

Even some activity is better than none, and health benefits increase proportionately to the time spent on physical activities.

How Much?

CDC recommends at least 150 minutes of moderate-intensity exercise or 75 minutes per week of vigorous-intensity activity for adults aged 65. Additionally, 2 days per week of muscle-strengthening activities and practices to improve balance are advisable.

Moderate and vigorous intensities reflect your efforts during exercises. For instance, moderate-intensity activity means you can talk but not sing during the training. It is only possible to utter a few words during vigorous practice.

For many seniors practicing this amount of fitness may not be possible due to bone and muscle stiffness, osteoarthritis, eye problems, or problems with nerve coordination. Simple tasks like eating, bathing, getting out of bed, and moving around the house may require assistance for many of you. Fear of losing balance and falls or injuries can make you feel more vulnerable.

Everyone loses mobility and body flexibility with age, but some lose them more than others.

We can have fitness in one area but lack it in another. A cyclist, for instance, may need more endurance for long-distance walking.

Being healthy is not the same as having fitness. You can be healthy without illnesses but lack strength, balance, or flexibility. On the other hand, you can be physically strong but have lifestyle illnesses due to heredity.

No matter what, reviewing CDC's guidelines, you can start fitness programs *anytime*, even with debilitating conditions like osteoarthritis. A*ny* amount of activity will help you find more stability and wellness. Physical activity will help you in performing daily self-care routines. Eventually, it will be possible for you to get noticeable improvement in daily functions.

Recent research suggests that even *half of the recommended level of exercise* can be enough to prevent injuries and falls and give other health benefits. This novel outlook would motivate many deconditioned and frail individuals to look forward to having an active life. They can start small exercise programs and continue them without getting too exhausted (Warburton et al., 2006).

Benefits of Physical Fitness

- Physical fitness keeps you active and independent.
- It improves body functions, including those who are overweight, obese, or weak.
- It reduces body weight, especially when combined with a regulated diet.
- It improves bone strength, muscle strength, and endurance.
- It improves the balance and flexibility of the body.
- It reduces the complications of lifestyle illnesses like type 2 diabetes or hypertension.
- It reduces the risk of dementia, anxiety, and depression.
- It boosts immune functions.

- It elevates mood and improves self-worth and social interactions.

Aerobic Activity

Aerobic activities like brisk walking, swimming, cycling, or dancing, are the best kind of exercises. They should be done on most days of the week. Any other activities like gardening, cleaning the house, or grocery shopping provide added benefits.

Aerobic activities are also known as endurance activities or cardio. In aerobic activities, we move the big muscles of our hands and feet repetitively for a considerable time, improving our strength.

The muscles use up glucose for readymade energy, which, in turn, improves metabolic functions.

Body fat is eventually utilized more to produce the energy required for exercising muscles. Thus, sustained aerobic exercise and a well-balanced diet reduce body weight.

Regular exercise improves heart and lung functions, producing better cardiovascular health.

Different types of activity, like walking the dog, bicycling to the local grocery, or dancing, enhance our body's adaptation to various postures. It improves our balance and flexibility.

CDC mentions that it is vital to maintain the *total amount* of activity recommended over the week instead of focusing on the duration of each activity period.

It means that even as little as *10 minutes of activity* at a stretch for three times a day is sufficient. Doing it five days a week completes the 150-minute recommendation for *moderate-intensity* exercise. You are encouraged to do more if you can.

Examples of Aerobic Activity

- Brisk walking

- Hiking
- Dancing
- Swimming
- Water aerobics
- Jogging or running
- Cycling: Stationary or outdoors
- Some yoga types
- Aerobic exercise classes
- Yard work such as raking or mowing
- Racquet sports or basketball

Muscle Strengthening

Muscle strengthening exercises include the following:

- Yoga or exercises using resistance bands or hand-held weights
- Workouts using body weight like pushups, pullups, planks, squats, or lunges
- Gardening
- Carrying grocery items
- Specific yoga postures and tai chi

Muscle training programs make the muscles work more than they are accustomed to, like climbing stairs, carrying weights, shoveling snow, etc. The exercises are for the muscles of the legs, hips, chest, back, abdomen, shoulders, and arms.

There is no fixed time for how long you should do these exercises. Repetitions must be continued until it is difficult for another one. Thus, repetitions of 10-12 per set in yoga postures are typically recommended. You are encouraged to do 2-3 of these sets.

But, it can be that exercise for you is a significant challenge. Your body is deconditioned and does not respond well to activity. You feel exhausted soon after.

Stay encouraged if this is the case with you. It is natural for your body to take time to adjust. When you do not exercise for a long time, muscles undergo disuse. They become emaciated and attenuated. The bones and joints also lose their ability to sense changes in posture and mobility.

It takes time for your body to respond to the benefits of exercise.

Muscles develop over time. Along with improving muscle power, endurance and balance are also built up.

It is always advisable to start with baby steps, particularly when your body is deconditioned. It means you start small repetitions but persevere in your attempts. Take a week or two to advance to the next level.

Gradually increase the number of repetitions, sets, and the time for exercise to achieve the desired counts.

Since the exercises are specific to a muscle or groups of muscles, several activities are needed to train them. However, the beauty of yoga is most postures involve many muscles. Hence, only a few yoga poses are enough to strength-train different body parts.

Balance Activities

Balance activities prevent falls and injuries like fractures. For proper balancing activity, we must be aware of the position of the joints of our body at rest and use this sense to guide joint motions during activities or movements.

Joint position sense or proprioception depends on agility, balance, and coordination. The capability to control the body during fast movements is agility. Balance keeps the body's line of gravity aligned with its support base. Coordination reflects harmonized action.

Like other features, body balance declines with aging. The chances of accidents increase with their deterioration, and you are scared to move around alone. Enforced incarceration diminishes muscle strength, coordination, and self-confidence. It creates a vicious cycle of disuse and immobility.

Balance activities can include practicing standing from a seated posture, using a wobble board, etc. Balancing is also improved by strengthening the back, stomach, and leg muscles.

Multi-component Activities

Multi-component activities blend aerobic training, muscle strength, adaptability, and coordination. Its examples are dancing, gardening, yoga, sports activities, and tai-chi. Yoga and tai chi are gaining popularity because they are inexpensive, engaging, and adaptable to individual needs and body types. Your attention is focused on molding and balancing your body here and now.

Yoga postures emulate the poses of birds and animals. These graceful movements flow with our form and can be compared to ballet. Like ballet, your body connects intimately with the mind as you breathe into different postures. That is why yoga is also a form of mindful meditation.

CDC considers yoga as light or moderate-intensity aerobic exercise. However, for seniors, these postures are considered moderate to vigorous-intensity activities. Some poses are also muscle-strengthening.

Warm-Up & Cool-Down

Warmups before aerobic activities increase the heart rate gradually, loosen the joints, and improve blood flow to the muscles, heating them up for the exercises. Warmup prepares the body to move with speed and agility, which is crucial for all training programs.

Cool-down allows the heart rate and breathing to settle back and muscles to return to their resting phase.

Typically a 5–10 minute period is adequate for warmup and cool-down.

Physical Fitness in Chronic Conditions

In the presence of comorbidities like type 2 diabetes mellitus, hypertension, a stroke, peripheral vascular diseases, or cancer, consult first with your doctor for the kind of physical activity suitable for you. Physicians agree that everyone, irrespective of the underlying conditions, must get some form of regular physical activity.

For **frail older adults**, regular physical activity helps with walking, gait coordination, and balance. Your quality of life gets satisfactory. You are encouraged to participate in any exercise that includes movement of different body parts at least thrice a week for half-an-hour sessions. It could be dusting the furniture or watering the plants. Guided physical rehabilitation programs that include exercises boost recovery after hip fracture.

Individuals with **functional limitations** who cannot perform everyday tasks benefit from regular exercise. Start with low-grade exercise routines as soon as you feel your usual self, and increase them gradually.

If you are recuperating from an **illness** like the common cold, or have recently **traveled**, rest adequately to recover.

Another aspect of physical fitness is its usefulness for individuals with a **disability**. Disablity mandates a structured and individualized exercise regimen under professional guidance. Activities are modified to suit individual needs, and supervision is recommended. You may need help with the movements you can carry out from a wheelchair or an arm ergometer.

Osteoarthritis is a debilitating condition among older people. The chronic condition causes stiffness, pain, and exhaustion. Beginning an activity is an extreme challenge. Even then, engaging with fitness routines and persevering improve joint and muscle stiffness, pain, and mobility. Low-impact yoga is particularly beneficial for individuals with osteoarthritis.

Type 2 diabetes includes exercise as an integral component of the treatment protocol—regular exercise benefits diabetics in countless ways. Heart conditions, blood lipids and sugar levels, bone and muscle health, nerve and gait coordination, and body weight are all improved following regular exercise programs.

Individuals with **high blood pressure** are benefitted from regular exercise, which reduces the risk of heart disease. Hypertensive individuals must consult with doctors before exercising regarding adjustment of the medication dosages.

Both **breast and colorectal cancers** benefit from regular physical activity, even after the diagnosis. Exhaustion is reduced, improving the quality of life. Further, the side effects of therapy take less toll on the patients.

Individuals suffering from **neurological problems** profit from physical fitness activity, particularly multi-component programs that include aerobic exercises, strength training, and coordination. Individuals with spinal cord injuries develop essential wheelchair skills, muscle strength, and upper extremity exercises.

Safety

- Start small and build your fitness routine gradually.
- Understand that you must be able to return to your program tomorrow. You can do that if you take adequate safety measures to protect your body from harm. Use protective gear, like good-quality soft-soled shoes and thick socks, and tools, like walking sticks, for exercise.

- Choose a safe environment with adequate heating and lighting provisions. Outdoor exercises in parks during the summer months can be relaxing.
- Consult your doctors if you are on medication for chronic conditions like type 2 diabetes or hypertension.
- Follow the rules and policies of an exercise program.

Real-Life Story

Ava was 87. She was busy all her life, working and raising two children. But after retiring from the postal services, Ava got increasingly sedentary. Old age and infirmity slowly overcame her once agile body, and she became a wheelchair user. Ava developed myriads of health issues, although she had no major illnesses.

Her doctor advised Ava to start a fitness routine. Skeptical at first, Ava agreed subsequently to start chair yoga. She was asked to base her functional level on the degree of exertion following a posture. Initially, she was doing chair yoga twice per week for 10 minutes. It gradually increased to 30 minutes per session. I included muscle-training yoga postures.

Ava agreed to thrice weekly classes as her strength and endurance increased. On two other days, Ava followed a video to step and walk in place for 10 minutes. She found enough power to walk upstairs to the roof with her daughter to enjoy beautiful sunsets.

Summary

- Exercise is beneficial for all seniors, irrespective of age or disability.
- Three Ten-minute sessions of daily activity are sufficient.
- Multi-component routines address aerobic exercise, muscle strengthening, and coordination.
- Yoga is a multi-component exercise.

The next chapter introduces you to the concept of chair yoga.

Chapter Two

The Concept of Chair Yoga

"Yoga is the destroyer of pain."

-Bhagavad Gita

Yoga is trendy in the US. Between 2010 - 2021, it grew by 63.8%. Of the 34.4 million yoga practitioners in America, women between 30 and 49 are the largest group (Smith, 2022). Undoubtedly the benefits of yoga account for its popularity.

You can practice yoga *asanas* anyplace and anytime per convenience. After learning them, you can do most of the asanas yourself. You do not need anything complicated to do the asanas or yoga postures. A mat, a chair, and a resistance band complete your list of equipment for yoga.

Why Yoga?

At first glance, the asanas can seem daunting. You may wonder how you can twist and turn your body into impossible angles and curvature that are the asanas. Even the calm, composed manner of the instructors seems forced and assuming. After all, how can they *imagine* that you will do this?

But they persist in their endeavor. They cajole you into trying a few asanas and see how you handle it. And to your surprise, you can fold your limbs and carry out the postures well. Of course, you wobble a lot and lose your balance several times, but the instructor's supportive hands guide you back to the asana. From there, you can manage on your own. And, it feels well. Your body senses the vibes of being thoroughly worked out, and your muscles feel stretched. You sweat with the effort and love the resulting warmness. In the end, you look forward to the next class.

Over the months, your stiffness eases, your pain is much less, and you feel a general sense of well-being. The postures that seemed challenging have become much easier. You can now water the plants, prune the herbs, and knit the woolen. You can venture to walk in the sunshine and plan for some grocery shopping or visit the cafe shop in your neighborhood pretty soon.

Thanks to yoga asanas, you have regained flexibility and strength to enjoy life's little pleasures. From pain reduction to the relief of joint stiffness, and muscle lengthening. yoga has helped countless individuals worldwide to gain health and wellness.

Breathwork

Yoga is intimately related to breath. The asanas are performed attuned to breathwork. For a beginner, it is tricky to concentrate on inhalation and exhalation while making conscious efforts to maintain balance. Once mastered, it becomes self-evident why the poses are dependent on breathing. It is easier to flow into the poses when we control and align breathing with the moves.

The essence of yoga is to breathe mindfully. Attention to breathing prevents external distractions, which can be dangerous during exercise. There are many scientific reasons to validate the unique technique of mind-body connection. The ancient sages of India used yoga to revive *prana*. Prana is energy. It must flow. Obstructed prana causes physical and mental disorders.

We learn to control breathing by consciously paying attention to it and slowing it down. The method induces a calming sensation. Additionally, breath work is the most straightforward approach to regulate the flow of prana, or vital energy, to all body parts. You may often hear your instructor asking you to breathe slowly and feel how your breaths reach the whole body, including the tips of your toes.

In pranayama, breath work includes inhalation, retention, and exhalation. Retention or holding of breath ensures better oxygen delivery to the body. It is soothing to the mind and reduces anxiety.

According to the yoga gurus, breathing produces vibration sounds. The sound of inhalation is 'So,' while that of exhalation is 'Ham.' As you go into the postures, you may repeat the mantra *soham* to connect breathing with the mind. It will draw your attention inward. It enables you to appreciate the effects of exercise on your body and mind.

Chair Yoga

For many of us, disability, significant osteoarthritis, and debilitating heart conditions can preclude conventional yoga postures. Standing for a considerable time may be challenging and sometimes impossible. You can still get the health benefits of yoga, including feel-good effects, by doing the postures from the safety of a chair.

Lakshmi Voelker-Binder has been credited with the intention of chair yoga techniques in 1982. An ardent believer and practitioner of yoga, Lakshmi taught many students. When one of her students could not participate in yoga classes owing to the untimely development of arthritis, Lakshmi created chair yoga postures for her to practice from the chair. Her mantra, "Get fit where you sit," has inspired countless people worldwide.

Benefits of Chair Yoga

You can do the same features of conventional yoga practice, including the asanas, meditation, and breathing techniques or pranayama from the chair. Most poses involve folding forward, bending backward, and twisting. All of them are adaptable for chair yoga. You can also use the chair as a support while executing the poses.

Chair yoga is the best exercise for seniors as it can loosen the joints, give the body pliability, and stretch the muscles, reducing chronic pain. Blood circulation to the joints is improved.

Chair yoga makes you less restless and anxious. Your stress-related blood pressure is reduced, and strength and balance are restored.

The benefits of consistent chair yoga practice are as follows:

- Maintain balance and body flexibility. These positive effects boost your confidence. Incidences of falls are considerably reduced.
- It improved muscle tone and strength, grip strength, and other physical measurements (Klempel et al., 2021).
- It boosts mood and reduces anxiety.
- You can manage chronic conditions like type 2 diabetes with chair yoga exercises. A randomized study of 10 patients, ranging from 49 - 77 years and with type 2 diabetes of more than 10 years, was conducted to see the effects of chair yoga on blood sugar levels and other related parameters. After 3 months of practice, individuals in the intervention group showed a reduction in fasting capillary blood glucose, heart rate, and diastolic blood pressure. The effects were not found in the control group (Mullur & Ames, 2016).
- It reduces chronic pain. A randomized pilot study found that an eight-week chair yoga practice effectively reduced pain, fatigue, and pain-related interference in osteoarthritis patients (Park et al., 2018).

Who can do Chair Yoga?

Anyone can do chair yoga, but it is especially beneficial in the following conditions:

- Individuals aged 65 years and older.

- Individuals with chronic health problems like dementia, type 2 diabetes, arthritis, or cardiac illnesses.
- Individuals with restricted mobility due to neurological problems like parkinsonism and spinal cord injuries.
- Individuals who spend long hours seated at home or office. Taking a small break from work to do a few seated yoga postures can relieve back and neck pain. It helps lessen the stress from the finger joints.
- Fifteen minutes of chair yoga in an office setup can boost physical health and reduce mental stress.

Individuals with chronic health problems and disabilities must take their physicians' advice before starting yoga.

Frequency & Duration of Sessions

You must aim for better physical and mental health through *consistent* practice. CDC recommends 30 minutes of training five days a week. It can be split into small components, each lasting 10 minutes over the day. First, practice twice weekly over a smaller amount of time and increase gradually.

Summary

- Statistics say American women between 30 and 49 practice yoga the most.
- Yoga boosts physical, mental, and emotional well-being.
- Yoga involves breathwork.
- Yoga gives the same benefit as mindful meditation.
- Practice it consistently for as long as you can without fatigue.

In the next chapter, we will discuss the best chair yoga postures.

Chapter Three

Chair Yoga Postures

"You were beautiful when young; you are still beautiful as old."

-Duo

Modern yoga asanas are modified to suit the individual requirements per age, or disability. Also called *accessible* or *adaptive* yoga, chair yoga is an essentially *low-impact exercise*.

Get energized by doing yoga in the cool morning hours before your day starts. However, you can do yoga anytime per convenience.

Practice the asanas every day. As little as a ten-minute session can prove helpful in setting the pace for the rest of the day.

The relevant question is to ask which chair is suitable for yoga poses. You can select any chair as long as it is stable and can bear your weight during the movements. Armless chairs are easy to practice with, and the back must support your trunk. The legs of the chair must be evenly positioned on the floor and should not wobble. Different companies have created suitable yoga chairs, but using them is optional.

Which gear must you wear for chair yoga? You do not need any special outfits, and regular clothes are just fine. However, avoid restrictive clothing and uncomfortable materials during exercise. Wear covered shoes with a proper fit.

Stay hydrated during the exercise. You do not need accessories besides the chair, a towel, or a resistance band. But, *avoid training immediately after meals*.

Warm-ups must precede all flexibility, strength training, and stretching postures. Hence, I have included the warm-up yoga poses before mentioning the others.

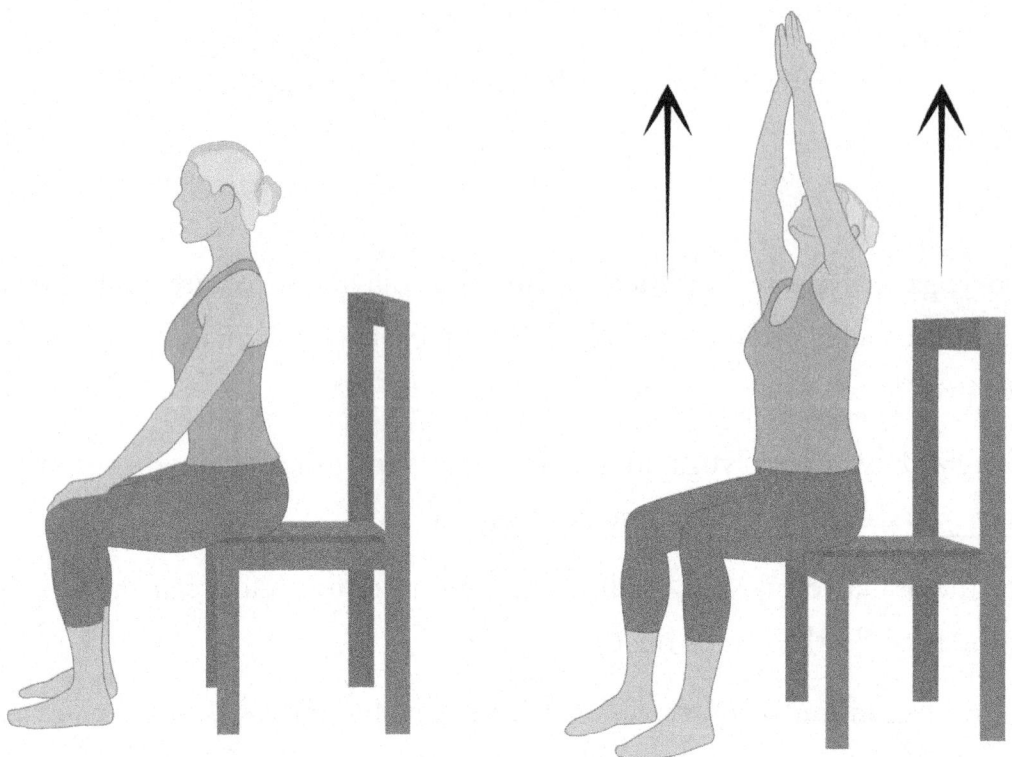

Overhead Stretch

Warm-Up

Overhead shoulder stretch, or *urdhahastasana*, gently opens your heart to the asana. Use this *warm-up* pose to start the training. Shoulder stretching helps to restore the balance between the sides of the body.

Muscles Stretched

All yoga postures stretch the muscles involved in making the moves. The arms, shoulders, and back muscles are stretched in this exercise.

Activity

- Place the chair on firm ground and sit up tall.
- Keep your shoulders back and down.
- Interlace the fingers of both hands.
- Raise your arms above your head toward the ceiling as far as possible. If this is difficult, raise both arms toward the ceiling without interlocking fingers.
- Remain in the asana for 10 - 20 seconds, appreciating the stretch in your arms, shoulders, and sides. Breathe slowly into the pose.
- Return to the original position.

Another variant:

- Lift both arms upward.
- Bend them at the elbows.
- Grasp the opposite elbows with each hand over your head.

Benefits

- Gives balance to the upper body.
- Reduces breathing problems.
- Strengthens abdominal muscles.

Contraindication

- Sprain and soreness in neck and shoulder regions.

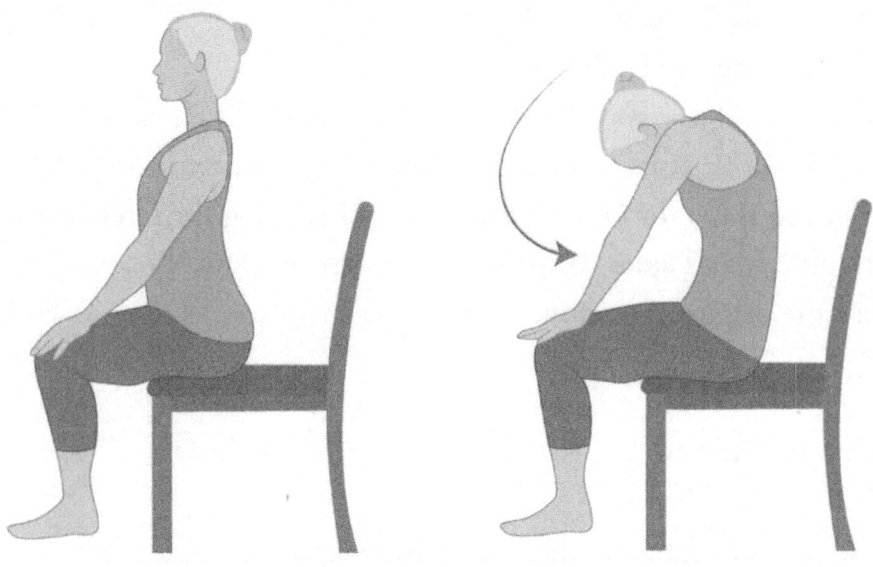

Cat-Cow Pose

Warm-Up Stretching

The yoga posture is a beautiful combination of forward and backward bends to stretch and relax the tight spots at the back, neck, and shoulder. You can use this versatile pose as a warm-up to other flexibility postures.

Method

- Sit tall at the chair's edge.
- Engage the core muscles by tightening the abdominals.
- Place both hands on your knees for support.

- Inhale and slowly arch your back, opening up your chest and lifting the chin for the cow pose.
- Hold the position for 3 - 5 breaths.
- As you exhale, fold forward, rounding your back, your chin touching the chest in a cat pose.
- Hold the position for 3 - 5 breaths.
- Release.

Benefits

- The soothing posture stretches the back.
- Calming to the mind.
- Stretches the abdominals.
- Opens the chest.

Contraindication

Recent abdominal surgery.

Injuries of the neck, shoulder, back, hips, or abdomen.

Neck Stretch

Flexibility

Poor postural practice and working long-term on laptops or phones can cause neck and shoulder muscle stiffness. If not addressed correctly, the muscles can become short and tight with time. Do gentle neck stretches to lengthen the neck muscles.

Remember, this is a relaxing exercise. Hence, let go of any tension during the posture and enjoy the *deep relaxation* it provides.

Method

- Sit tall in your chair without the support of its back.

- Lift your chin so that the crown of your head moves toward the ceiling.
- Using the sides of the chair to support your right hand, slowly lift your left hand and touch the left temple.
- Inhale, and gently dip your head toward the left side as you exhale. Your left ear points toward the left shoulder.
- Keep the right shoulder level throughout the exercise. Keep your back straight.
- Breathe in and out for 10 - 20 seconds.
- Release.
- Repeat the movement on the other side.

Add some challenge to the asana by moving your neck against resistance.

Benefit

Do the exercise mindfully to get all the benefits.

- Releases stress.
- Reduces neck pain.
- Relaxation of the whole body.

Contraindication

- Avoid neck stretches after neck, spine, or shoulder injuries, inflammation, or surgeries.
- Reduce acute pain with ice, rest, painkillers, neck collar, and heat. Then do some gentle stretches and avoid bad posture.

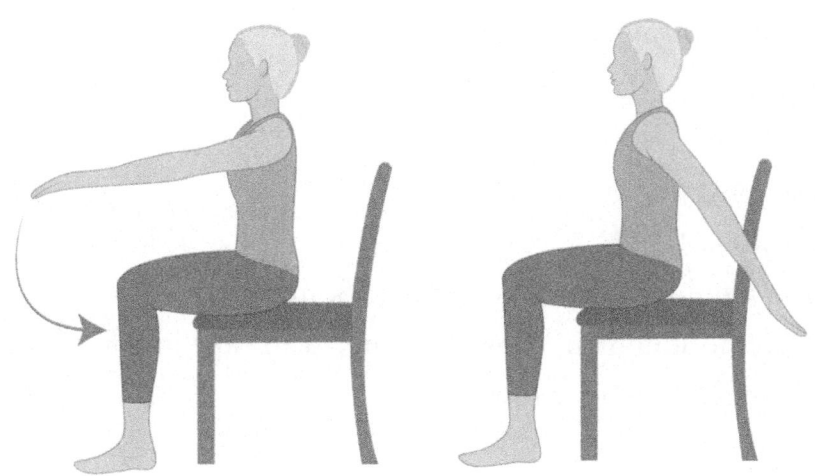

Reverse Arm Hold

Stretching

Reverse arm hold, or *paschim namaskarasana*, acts on the muscles of the arm and abdomen.

Method

- Sit upright in a chair without the support of the back.
- Inhale deeply, straighten both arms at your sides, forming a low and wide angle.
- As you exhale, bend your arms slightly at the elbows and reach them behind your back.
- Arch your back to feel the stretch in your shoulders.

- Hold the pose for 10 - 20 seconds.
- Release.

In a more challenging version of the exercise, you may fold your arms behind your back in a gesture of *namaste in reverse*.

Benefit

- Improves posture
- Relieves stress
- Stretches shoulder joints and upper back muscles.
- Opens up the abdomen, allowing more air to flow into the lungs.
- Releases spinal muscle tension.

Contraindication

- Spinal problems
- High blood pressure

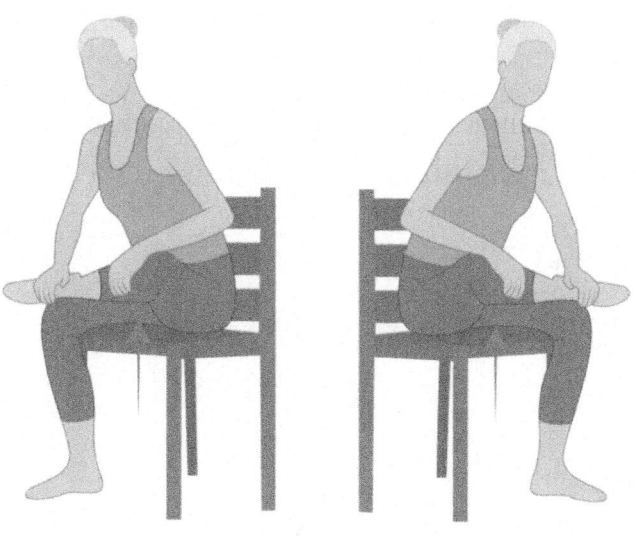

Chair Pigeon

Flexibility

Pigeon pose or kapotasana is popularly used to stretch the hips and lower back muscles.

Method

- Sit straight with your back away from the chair's back.
- Slowly lift your left ankle and rest it on your right knee or thigh. Use your hand to guide the left ankle to this position.
- Inhale and bend forward on exhalation, pushing the left knee downward with the left hand and lifting the foot upward with the right hand.
- Hold the position for 10 - 20 seconds.
- Release hold.

- Return to the original position.
- Repeat the asana with the opposite leg.
- For individuals with mobility problems, another modification involves the following:
- Cross your feet at the ankles, your hands resting on the knees.
- Inhale and fold forward, pushing down slightly on the knees until you feel a stretch in your hips.
- Hold for 3 - 5 breaths.
- Release the pressure of your hands as you exhale.

Benefit

- Boosts flexibility of hip joints.
- Stretches hip muscles, hamstring, and calf muscles.
- Improves posture.
- Reduces lower back pain.

Contraindication

- Avoid doing the exercise in ankle, foot, and hip joint injuries or after surgery involving these regions.

Forward Fold

Stretching

In Sanskrit, this asana is called uttanasana; you bend forward as much as attainable. Let your hands rest on the floor as you fold over your legs, if possible. Allow the head to drop down.

Method

- Sit tall with your back away from the chair's back. Your knees should touch, and your feet firm on the floor.

- Inhale, and as you exhale, gently bend forward, feeling how your back lengthens one vertebra after another.
- Lean forward as much as you can without exerting yourself.
- Hold the position for 3 - 5 breaths.
- Release.

Benefits

- Stimulation of the liver and kidneys.
- Better digestion.
- Reduction of stress.
- Reduction of blood pressure.
- Relieves lower back pain.

Contraindication

- Lower back or neck injuries.
- Glaucoma.
- Uncontrolled blood pressure.
- Spinal deformities and osteoporosis.

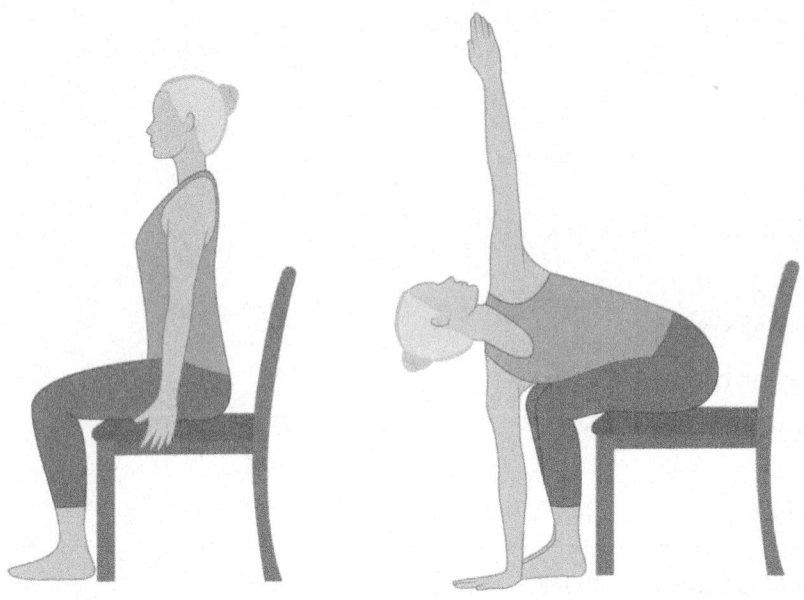

Extended Side-Angle

Stretching

The pose, called *parsvakonasana* in Sanskrit, is an extension of the chair forward fold. It is a modification of the warrior pose.

Method

- Hold your position after folding forward.
- Gently lower the fingertips of your left hand to the floor, just outside the left foot. If this is challenging, use a block to rest your fingertips or lower them to the left knee.

- Inhale and twist to the right, raising the right arm slowly toward the ceiling, your gaze looking up.
- Hold the position for 3 - 5 breaths.
- Exhale as you lower the right arm and come back to rest.
- Repeat the posture on the opposite side.

Benefit

- Stretching exercise for the leg, hip muscles, and hamstring.
- Opens up chest and shoulders.
- Relieves body stiffness.

Contraindication

- Injuries to shoulder.
- High blood pressure.
- Vertigo.

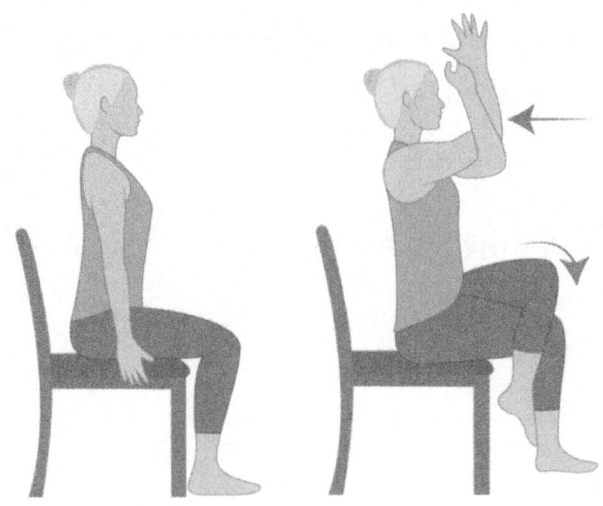

Eagle-Arms

Stretching

In Sanskrit, the posture is called *garudasana*.

Method

- Sit upright on the edge of a chair, ensuring your balance.
- Lift your right leg and cross it over the left thigh. If possible, wrap it around the left calf.
- Cross your left arm over the right arm at the elbow. Bend the elbows and bring your palms to touch each other in front of you.
- Gradually lift the elbows. Drop the shoulders away from the ears.
- Hold the posture for 3 - 5 breaths.

- Repeat on the opposite side.

Benefit

- Improves attention.
- Improves blood circulation to the arms.
- Good for digestion and elimination processes.

Contraindication

- Injuries of knee, elbow, wrist, or shoulder.
- Problems with balance.

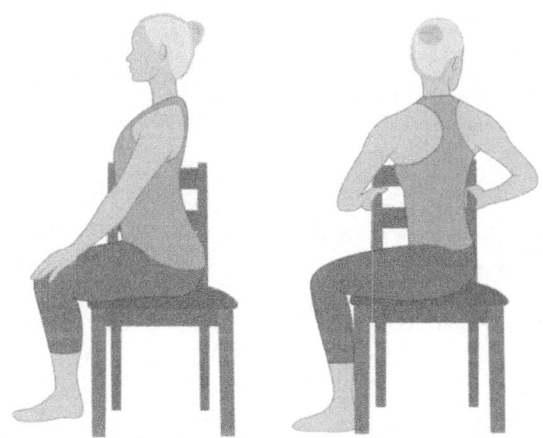

Spinal Twist

Stretching

This asana is called *ardha matsyandresana* in Sanskrit. If you do it regularly, you will lose your balance.

Method

- Sit sideways, facing left on the chair without touching its back.
- Inhale and lengthen your spine.
- As you exhale, slowly twist your body to the left side, your face toward the left. Hold to the back of the chair for support.
- Inhale and lengthen your spine, and twist to the left on exhalation.
- Repeat the movement 3 - 5 times.
- Turn to your right and carry out the asana on this side 3 - 5 times.

Benefit

- Lengthening of the spine.
- Improves flexibility.
- Improves back pain.

Contraindication

- Obesity.
- Knee problems.
- Injuries in the tail bone.
- Individuals unable to coordinate body movement with breathwork.

Seated Mountain

Joint Stiffness

The mountain pose, or tadasana, stabilizes the core. This pose is frequently used in yoga as a baseline before starting another asana. To engage the core, inhale and draw your belly button toward the spine. There are no special contraindications to seated mountain pose.

Method I

- Sit tall on the edge of the chair and engage your core.
- Keep your knees parallel to the ground over the ankles. There should be a small gap between them.
- Inhale deeply. Upon exhalation, roll your shoulders downward.
- Actively using your abdominal muscles, press your arms down at your sides.
- Hold the pose for 3 - 5 breaths.

Method II

- Inhale deeply, and as you exhale, fix your body weight firmly on your tailbone on the chair.
- Inhale.
- Exhale, roll your shoulders down your back, engage the core, and raise the arms to your sides, opening up your heart.
- Hold the position for 3 - 5 breaths.
- Release and relax.

Benefit

- Engages core.
- Corrects posture and stiffness.
- Establishes mind-body connection.

The following five yoga postures are challenging for beginners. However, as you practice and gradually get habituated to doing yoga and gain strength, and mobility, you can attempt these postures under the right guidance.

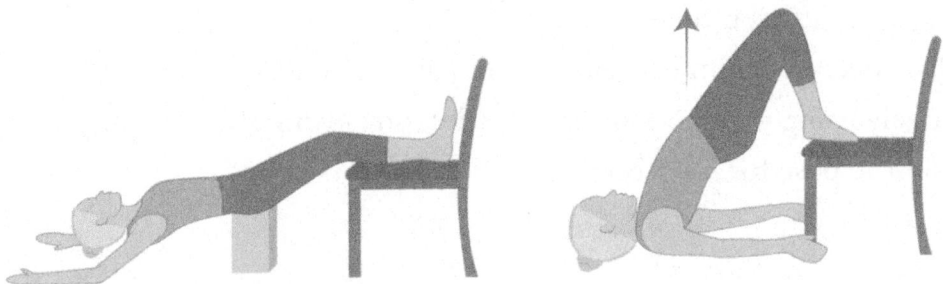

Bridge Pose

Stretching

Also called setubandha sarvangasana, the bridge pose is to hold your body in an arch to resemble a bridge. You need towels, a mat, and a *low deep chair* as a prop in this asana.

Method

- Take a stable chair on which you will rest the lower part of your body.
- Place a folded towel on the edge of the chair to support your back and limbs.
- Place another folded towel on the mat to support your head, neck, and upper body.
- Lie down on the mat, your neck, and body supported by towels.
- Slowly lift your body from the waist, one leg first and then the other, to rest on the chair's seat. Your lower half of the body forms an angle with the floor.
- Feel the stretch at your back as you relax into the pose.

Benefit

- Lowers blood pressure
- Relieves backache.
- Prevents varicose veins.

Contraindication

- Backache
- Injury and recent surgery of the back, neck, and limbs.

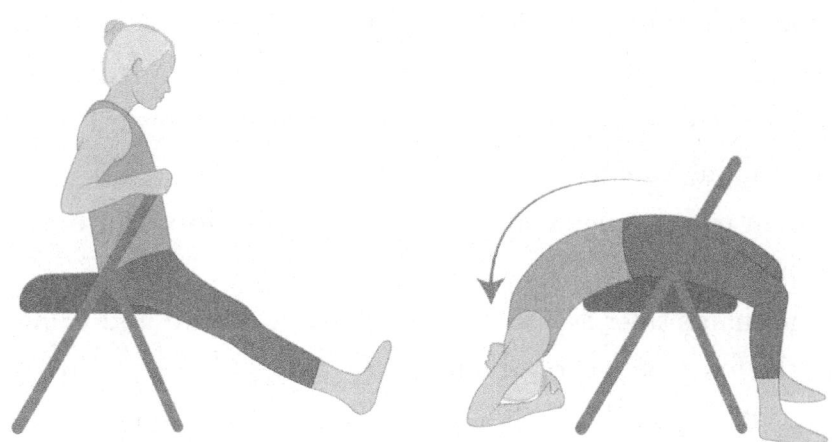

Inverted Staff Pose

Stretching

This asana is called viparita dandasana in Sanskrit. We will discuss it in two parts; the second is more challenging. For the asana, you need a *mid-back chair* with a back only in its upper half, a mat, and folded towels on the carpet to support your head.

Method

- Do the warm-up asanas first.
- Sit tall facing the back of the chair, passing your feet through the gap in its back.
- Hold the back of the chair for better support.
- As you slide your hands down the sides of the chair, inhale, and as you exhale, incline backward from your waist, your head tilted toward the ceiling.
- Stretch as far as possible.
- If you want to challenge yourself, slide your hips forward to rest on the edge of the chair.
- Hold the chair's sides as you tilt your body backward and bring your head to rest on the folded towel on the mat.
- In full posture, your body should rest on the chair, your legs straight out, and your head resting on the towel.

Benefit

- Stimulates hormone action.
- Improves digestion, heart and lung functions.
- Improves spinal flexibility.
- Reduces backache.

Contraindication

- Migraine

- Vertigo
- Acute spinal injury.

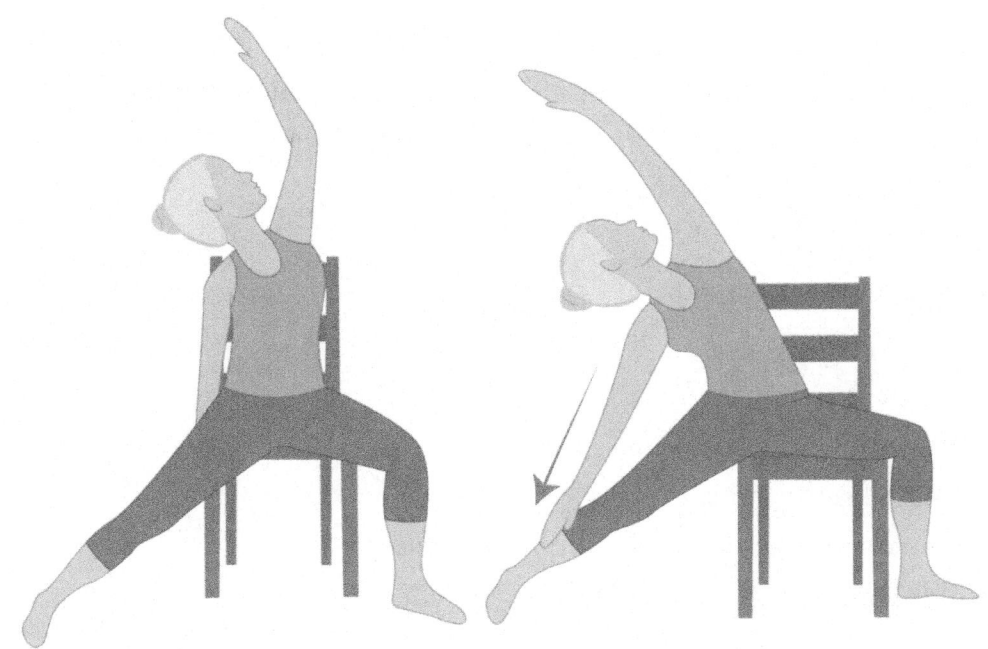

Reverse Warrior

Strengthening & Flexibility

Several asanas in yoga involve forward and backward folds, but side bends are less common. Reverse warrior is more a side bender than a back fold. Indeed, you are discouraged from bending backward to make a full-length spinal extension.

Method

- Sit sideways on the edge of a chair, balancing yourself well. Your left knee is bent at a right angle, over the ankle, and your right leg is swung back. Adjust your position to align your trunk with the right hip.

- Inhale and raise both arms, your left arm facing you and your right arm held backward.
- Exhale.
- Raise your left arm above your head as you bend toward the right side, your right arm sliding down the right leg. Look up to follow the movement of the left arm above.
- Hold the pose for three breaths.
- Release and relax.
- Repeat on the other side.

Benefit

- Opens up the rib muscles.
- Strengthens the arms.
- Improves mobility and flexibility of the back.
- Builds core strength and balance.
- Stretches the thigh.
- Opens up the hip.
- Energizes the body.

Contraindication

- Problems balancing.
- Injuries to hips, knees, back, or shoulders.
- You should feel a stretch in your groin, thighs, and sides, but no pain. If you feel pain, abandon the pose.

Single-Leg Stretch

Stretching

Also called janusirasana in Sanskrit, single-leg stretch, as the name suggests, is a stretching yoga pose. You can do it seated in a chair.

Method

- Sit tall near the edge of the chair. Ensure your balance.
- Stretch out your right leg, your heel planted on the floor, and the toes looking up.
- Place both hands on the outstretched leg.
- Inhale, elevating the spine, and on exhalation, fold over your right leg, sliding your hands down it with body movement.
- Move down the leg to grasp the right ankle or the back of the right calf. Otherwise, bend down as far as possible without straining your back or exerting yourself.
- Take five deep breaths, going deeper with each breath.
- Inhale and rise.
- Repeat the movement with the left leg.

Benefit

- Stimulates digestion and elimination.
- Strengthens lung functions.
- Improves blood sugar.
- Strengthens and tones thigh and calf muscles.
- Restorative.

Contraindication

- High blood pressure.
- Asthma.
- Knee injury.

Savasana

Joint stiffness

Savasana is a profoundly relaxing or resting pose. All yoga training end with savasana, which establishes a deep connection between the body and our inner spirit. Typically, savasana or corpse pose is done by lying on the ground. However, we may use a chair to end our practice session with this restorative posture (Pizer, 2022).

Method

- Sit on the chair with your eyes closed.
- Keep your hands on your lap.
- Clear your mind of thoughts and let go of any tension, even thoughts about breathing.
- Swallow once to remove the anticipation in your throat.
- Allow your body to go limp, removing all vestiges of tension.
- Breathe evenly and effortlessly as you relax in this resting pose.
- To release the posture, deepen your breathing, curl your fingers and toes, and reach up with your hands, giving a final stretch to your body.

Benefit

- Full body relaxation.
- Mindful awareness of the body.
- Allows evaluation for any muscle tension which is consciously released.
- Rejuvenation of the body and the mind.

Summary

- Use a stable chair without an armrest to do chair yoga.
- The chair should be firm on the ground and able to carry your weight.
- Begin postures with a warm-up, and end them with a cool-down.

- Gradually mold into the asanas without exerting yourself.
- To begin with, select three to four asanas, and repeat each asana two to three times. Gradually increase the frequencies and repetitions.

Chapter Four

More Chair Yoga Postures

In this chapter, I will present the celebrated posture of Surya Namaskar. If you are wondering whether you can do it from a chair, let me assure you that you can enjoy doing this beautiful pose that opens up the body from the safety of a chair.

I have included some more asanas that are perfect for treating low back pain, joint stiffness, and pain associated with osteoarthritis. Some of the asanas use the cair as a prop. The last two asanas are *ujjayi* asana, a type of *pranayama*, and *chair meditation*.

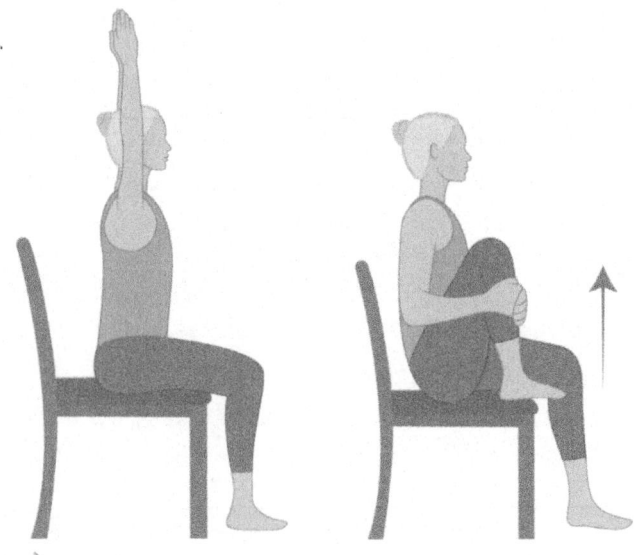

Surya Namaskar

Warm-Up, Opening-Up

Surya, or the sun, is our life-giving force. In the pose, we are grateful to this indomitable energy source that vitalizes all living beings.

It has 12 steps or sequences.

Method

- Sit tall on a chair; your back away from the chair's back. Hold your feet close together.
- Bring your hands to your chest, fold them, and connect the palms in a *namaste* pose.
- Breathe slowly, relaxing your body.
- Stretch your arms backwards as far as possible, bending your body back with the arms. Your feet must be planted on the ground.
- Exhale and gently bring your hands down, resting them on your thighs.
- Now fold forward, trying to touch your toes with your hands.
- Holding the position, exhale, and stretch one arm toward the ceiling.
- Hold the pose for 5 - 10 seconds—a fantastic twist to your body.
- Release and rest for a few seconds.
- Repeat the movements on the other side.
- Fold one leg and lift it on the chair. Support the leg with both hands.
- Hold for 5 - 10 seconds.
- Release the leg, bend forward, sliding your hands down your legs.
- Now fold the other leg and lift it up on the chair, holding it with both hands for support.
- Maintain the posture for 5 - 10 seconds.
- Release the leg on the ground.
- Complete the asana by repeating the forward fold and, finally, the backward fold.

Benefit

- Strengthens spine.
- Improves mobility.
- Lengthening of different muscle groups.
- Stimulates prana or life force.

As you practice Surya namaskar regularly, you will appreciate the lengthening of your backbone and loosening up the joints.

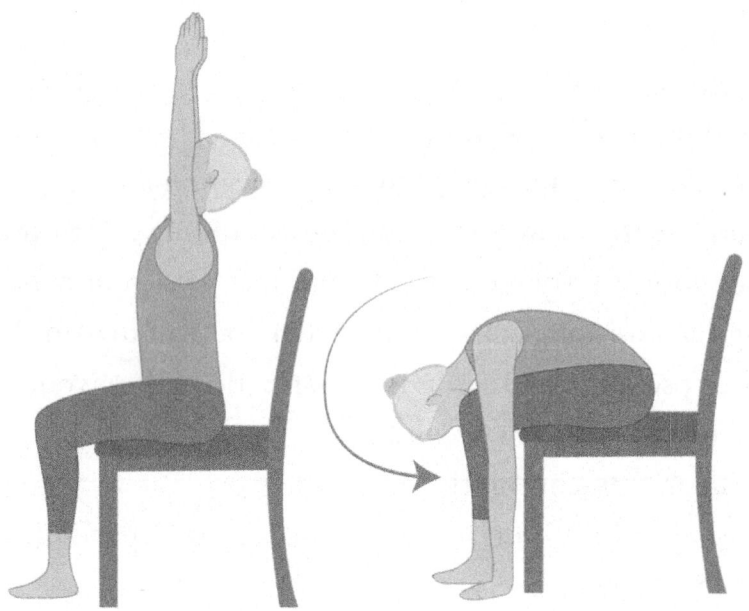

Chair Pose

For Low Back Pain

The chair pose is called *utkatasana* in Sanskrit. When done standing, it folds the body like a chair, hence the name.

Select a stable chair with its feet firmly placed on the ground in the chair version of the chair pose.

Method

- Sit upright without touching the back of the chair. Rest your feet on the floor.

- Exhale and lean forward until your shoulders cross half of the thighs or as much as is comfortably possible.
- Inhale and lift both arms over your head, palms facing each other at shoulder-width apart.
- Hold the pose for 5 - 10 seconds.

Benefit

- Strengthens the leg, ankle, lower back, and core muscles.
- Strengthens shoulders and upper back.

Contraindication

- Significant lower back problems when it must be done under medical supervision.
- Recent injuries.
- Uncontrolled blood pressure.

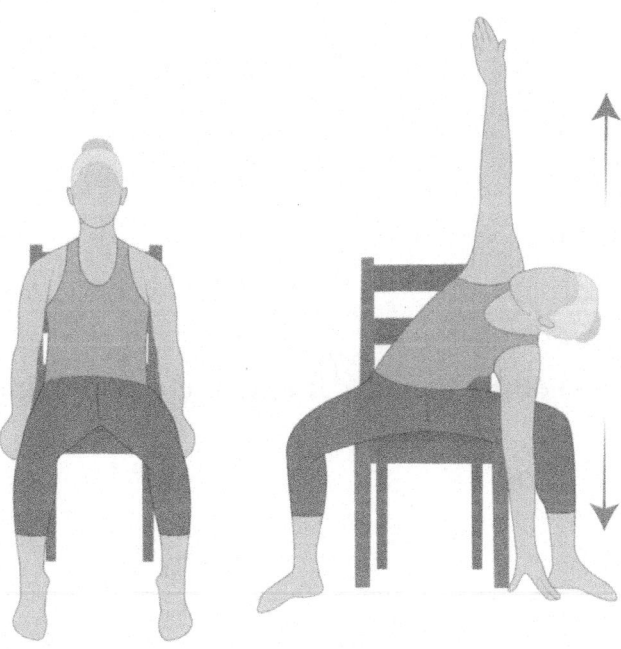

Triangle Pose

For Backache

The triangle pose or trikonasana is an excellent posture to relieve backache, neck pain, and sciatica.

Method

- Sit upright, your feet clear of the chair's edge, and pointed outward.
- Inhale and raise your arms parallel to the floor.
- Hold and exhale.
- Inhale again and reach your right hand toward the floor to touch the inside of the right thigh. Simultaneously, lift the left arm toward the ceiling as you gaze up.
- Hold the position for 5 - 10 seconds.
- Release and repeat on the other side.

Benefit

- Strengthen the core, shoulders, and back muscles.
- Stretches the groin.
- Relieves back pain.

Contraindication

Acute pain and trauma of the shoulder and neck joints and muscles.

Chair Downward Dog

For Backpain

The downward dog yoga pose is a basic asana for many Ashtanga and Vinyasa practices. It is of intermediate challenge.

Method

You can do the posture with the support of the back or the cahir seat. You can also use the help of a countertop or table.

- Stand tall, inhale deeply, and raise your arms above your head.
- As you exhale, place both hands on the back of the chair or any other stable object. If your knees bend, do not worry.
- Push yourself back slowly until your back lengthens, parallel to the ground. Feel a stretch in the shoulders, hamstrings, and calves.
- Hold the position for 5 - 10 seconds.
- Slowly walk forward and once you approach the chair, inhale, and straighten the back, raising your arms toward the ceiling.

Benefit

- Strengthens the shoulder, lower back, legs, ankles, feet, and core muscles.
- Stretches the lower body.
- Improves blood circulation.

Contraindication

- Injury of arms, shoulders, and back.
- High blood pressure.
- Vertigo.

The following yoga postures benefit osteoarthritis, a degenerative bone condition occurring with aging. It destroys the protective cartilage at the bone ends that form the joints, resulting in increased friction between bone surfaces with movement and pain.

The best treatments for osteoarthritis include a healthy diet, regulated body weight, and regular exercise.

Yoga allays osteoarthritis-induced joint stiffness and pain. It restores mobility and flexibility. Use the following yoga movements for each body part to improve bone health. The neck and the torso exercises include neck movements, cat-cow, and spinal twist postures described in chapter one (Dr. Moonaz, 2019).

Contraindications for these exercises are acute injury to the body parts.

Feet & Ankles

Warm-Up

Method

- Sit upright on a stable chair.
- Your feet should be under your toes.
- Spread your toes and place them on the floor. Press your heels.
- Lift the toes and wiggle them a little.
- Lift your heels, and alternately lift the toes.
- Raise your feet a few inches from the ground and move your ankles up and down. Make circular motions first in one direction and then in another.
- Turn the soles of the feet toward each other.
- Turn them out and feel the squeeze in the thighs.
- Place your feet on the ground heel first and then lower the toes on the ground one by one.
- Take one foot forward and the other backward and reverse in a seated march.

Benefit

- The movements are grounding and relaxing.
- They increase blood flow to the ankles, calves, and feet.
- Raised leg movements alternately open and squeeze the groin.

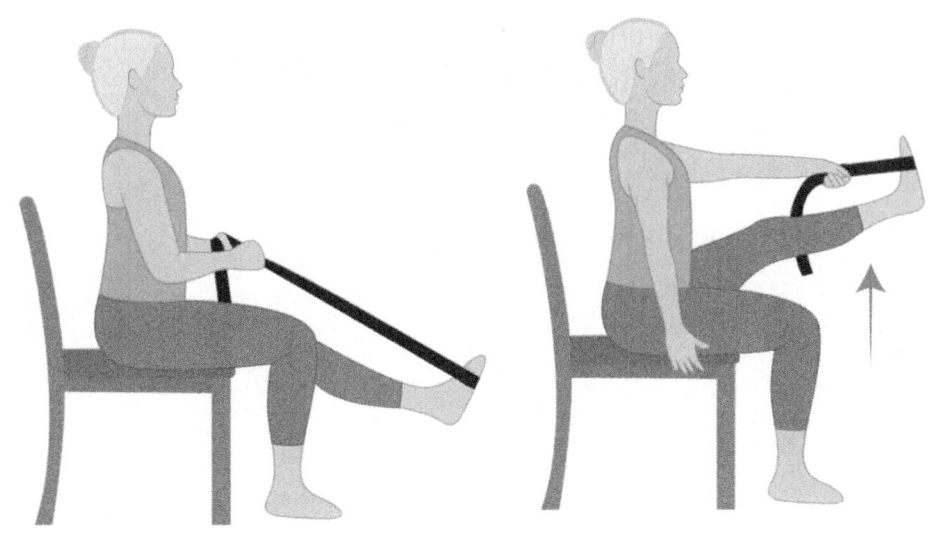

Leg

Hamstring Stretch

Use a resistance band or a hand towel to do this asana, also called utthita hasta padangusthasa.

Method

- Hook a towel or a band around your left foot, holding its ends with your left hand. Your other hand can be on the edge of the chair for better support.
- Lift your right leg, keeping your back tall. Don't worry if the knee bends.
- Hold the pose, wiggling your toes for better blood flow to the calves.
- Loosening the tension on the band will make your hip muscles work more.
- Release and repeat on the other side.

- You can do the asana without a band.
- Lift the legs one by one and then both together.
- Draw big circles first on one side, then on the other.
- Spread your arms out for better balance.

Benefit

- Stretches and strengthens the leg muscles.

Shoulder

Warm-Up

Method

- Raise your shoulder a little and gently roll them one way and then in a reverse direction.
- Move your arms forward and then slide them backwards.
- Make circles with your arms, first in one direction and then reverse.
- Try making swimming movements with your arms.
- You can also do shoulder stretches with a band or towel.
- Use a band to spread your arms at your sides, front, and above your head.

Benefit

- Opens up the shoulder and strengthens the arm muscles.
- Improves blood flow to the exercising parts.

Fingers & Wrists

Warm-Up

Method

- Sit on a chair and spread your arms in front of you.

- Spread the fingertips, and bring them together. Don't worry if they don't touch.
- Repeat the movement as if you are squeezing a ball.
- Imagine playing the piano.
- Roll the wrists in and out.
- Flap your hands in upward and downward motions at the wrist. Do doggy paddle.
- Make a fist, and open up with the thumb inside the fist and then outside.
- Shake your arms.

Benefit

- The movements allow joint lubrication and reduce stiffness and pain.

High Alter Side Leans

Stretching

Method

- Sit upright.
- Lift your arms, interlacing your fingers in front of you.
- Raise the arms toward the ceiling.
- Inhale.
- Exhale and tilt your arms to the right.
- Inhale to come back to the center.
- Repeat the movement three times on each side, flowing with your breath.

Benefit

- Stretches the spine and the shoulders.

Contraindication

- Injury to shoulder and neck.
- Vertigo.

Hip Circles

Flexibility

Method

- Sit tall.
- Make 5 circular hip movements on the seat without moving your upper body.
- Repeat the movements counterclockwise.

Benefit

- Releases and relaxes the hip muscles.

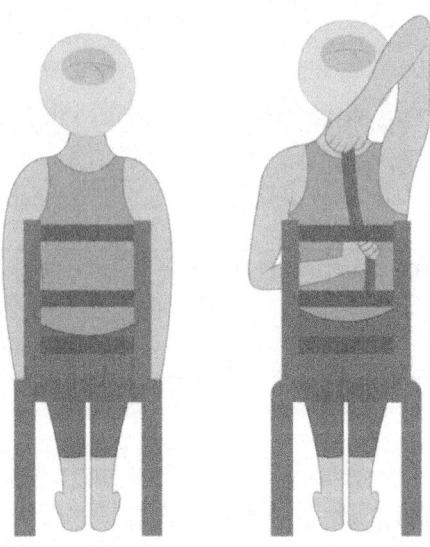

Cow-Face Pose

Stretching

Also called gomukhasana in Sanskrit, the cow-face pose is another beautiful way to challenge your body.

Method

- Sit upright on a stable chair without touching its back.
- Cross one leg over the other, or keep them together if it's easier for you.
- Shift your weight to sit on the tailbone.
- Raise one hand *toward the ceiling*, bend it at the elbow, and take it to your back. The hand is directed downward. You can hold a towel in this hand to complete the asana.
- Raise the other arm *to your side*, bend it at the elbow, and take it to your back. This hand is directed upward to catch the towel.
- Grasp both hands, interlocking the fingers. Use a towel or a resistance band if it's challenging to hold the hands behind your back.
- Hold the pose for 5 -10 seconds.
- Release and relax.
- Repeat the posture switching the arms on the other side.

Benefit

- Whole body stretching.
- Flexibility and posture.
- Grounding and calming.

Contraindication

- Acute pain in the neck, shoulder, arms, and back.
- Injury to muscles.

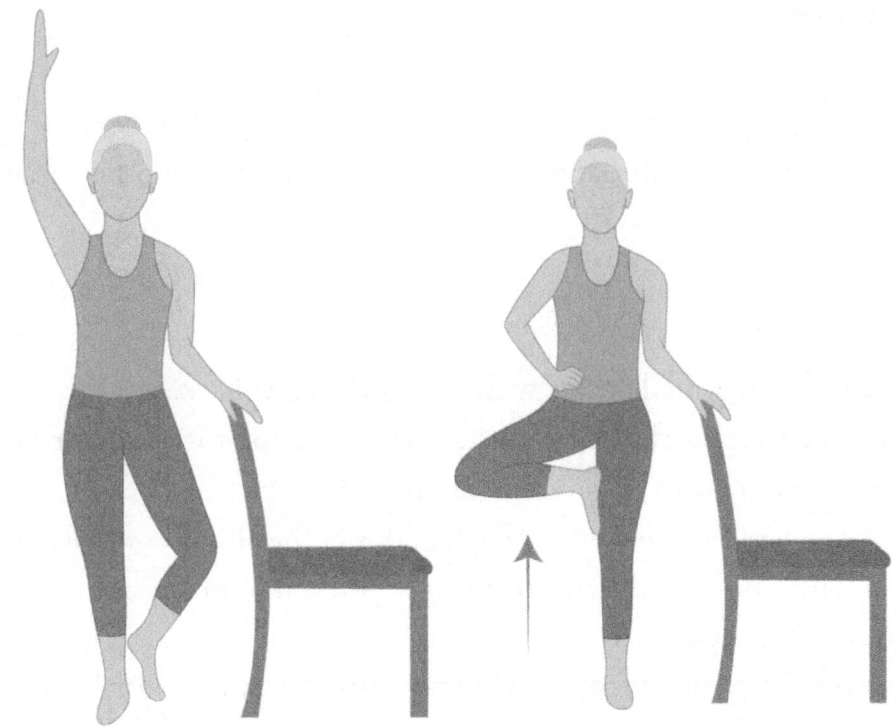

Tree pose

Stretching

The tree pose, or Vrksashana mimics the tree. It is done standing. You can use a chair to do the pose.

Method

- Stand tall in the mountain pose behind a stable chair.
- Hold the chair's back with both hands.
- Shift your weight on the right leg and gently lift the left leg from the floor.
- Bring the left leg to rest on the inner side of the right thigh, or keep it lifted if it's easier for you.
- Hold the pose for 5 - 10 breaths.
- Release and repeat on the other side.

Benefit

- Stretches the leg muscles.
- Opens the hip and stretches the inner thigh.
- Helps in balance and posture.

Contraindication

- Injury to knee, foot, and ankle.
- Vertigo.

Ujjayi Breathing

Ujjayi or ocean breath is a pranayama yoga posture, calming to the mind.

Method

- Sit upright, your feet on the floor. Close your eyes.
- Place your hands on your waist.
- Inhale deeply through the nose, making the sounds of the ocean as air passes through a constricted throat to expand your sides and the abdomen.
- Hold for six seconds.
- Exhale slowly.
- Repeat for ten breaths.

Benefit

- Therapeutic for thyroid problems.
- Improves oxygen saturation.
- Lowers blood pressure.
- Reduces anxiety.

Chair Meditation

Several studies have shown how meditation relieves knee joint pain and stiffness (Selfe & Innes, 2013). Mindful meditation forms an essential component of pain therapy for chronic arthritis.

Method

- Choose a straight-back stable chair.
- Roll a blanket on the seat to sit tall and comfortably.
- Keep your thighs parallel to the floor. Your feet should be resting on the floor.
- You can slip a meditation or any cushion between your back and the chair's back. You must not slouch, or relax back on the chair.
- Place your hands on your thighs, palms facing up. Roll your shoulders back, your head aligned with the shoulders. Lift up your chin.
- Release all tensions from your body.
- You may close your eyes, and when you are ready, start by becoming aware of your breaths flowing in and out of your body.
- Feel where the air movement is the most, nose, chest, or belly? Fix your attention to only one location.
- Focus on this area and notice the physical sensation of your breath on the body. Get curious about each breath, and how each sensation is different from the other.
- Each time you notice your mind shifting away, gently bring your attention back to breathing.
- When you are ready, let go of your attention on your breath, and slowly open your eyes.

Benefit

- Eases arthritis pain.

Conclusion

Old age problems can incapacitate us. We always considered retirement an ability to do all we never had time for in our youth. Taking vacations to far-away places, picking up hobbies, or spending time with our grandchildren were some of the many dreams we reserved for our post-work years.

All that could still be yours, despite those aches and pain, intolerable at times. The trick is how to look at the glass: half-full or half-empty? However you look at it, the glass always contains the same amount of water.

But perspectives matter. Consider your glass half-empty. It immediately creates a panic mode of action, spurred by an intense fear of loss of privilege, anxiety, deprivation, and defeat. Loss and fear are exceedingly negative emotions.

Now consider your glass is half-full. The thought of it relaxes you, and you think there is still a lot to finish. You feel thankful and confident.

When we face what we have with a positive outlook, we also allow ourselves to look for suitable options even when the experience is unwelcoming. Our fear is replaced by courage and spirit. We renew our faith in our choices and actions.

It is our attitude that is the real game changer. So, with that attitude, let us embrace regular chair yoga practices described in this book to show how we can fulfill our golden days and make ourselves proud.

Balance & Fall Prevention Program

Improve Your Core Strength & Regain Your Coordination to Remain Independent.

Introduction

Anna did not even understand how she fell down. She was wearing her usual pumps: durable shoes without heels, the day was bright and sunny, and the road was dry and squeaky clean. One moment Anna was walking down the road; a couple was ahead of her, and she was thinking about what she would cook for lunch today. The next moment, she was on the ground, her groceries having spilled all over the sidewalk from the torn paper bag, and more embarrassingly, two young adults, men of her son's age, were trying to pull her up.

They were concerned and repeatedly asked if Anna could stand, how she was feeling, and whether she could go home on her own or if they needed to call someone for her.

Anna was furious with herself for letting others down for no reason at all. She did not want to inform her son, who lived in another part of the country and would, in all probability, be asleep by now. And what would he think? That her mother was incapable of walking in the street at 60?

Falls are common concerns for women in Anna's age group between 50 years - 70 years and above. They mostly happen suddenly, without apparent reasons, and this surprise element scares us who belong to this age bracket.

The period is vulnerable and is one of the major life transitions for us. Our bodies become frail, our eyesight diminishes, our hearing acuity is much less than it used to be, and our balance falters. We face challenges from home and family life, too. If we have already retired, we have more time on our hands than necessary. Our careers kept us busy and engaged, and suddenly there was a void.

At home, our children have already left the nest or are leaving. Even if they stay close by, they have their lives and career to juggle. We do not want to overwhelm them with our weaknesses.

Falls and accidents can happen in many ways.

Another example would be of a lady who visited me a while back. Her name was Klara, and her story shows us how devastating falls can be, particularly when it comes to shattering our self-confidence.

When Klara came to me, she was worried. The 50-plus lady was afraid. She recently had a fall during exercise at home. But more than that, what scared her was what her daughter would say when she heard about her accident. Would she prevent Klara from using the treadmill she recently bought?

Klara loved to exercise indoors, and using the treadmill for brisk walks was her forte. Her husband presented Klara with a treadmill, and since then, she has walked at home. For privacy, she shut the door while exercising. It was Klara's habit to listen to music as she walked. Today was no exception until someone knocked on the door. Klara turned around and fell. Since the treadmill was operating, she was thrown against the handrail, and she tumbled, her foot caught in the space between the running deck and the roller.

Klara was afraid. She did not know why she fell. Although she had hypertension and was on medications, her blood pressure was controlled. She had no other physical ailments, and her mental acumen was sharp. She also took her Vitamin D and calcium supplements regularly. Was she then suffering from some neurological conditions? Would that prevent her from walking? Her husband was certainly skeptical. Was this related to Klara approaching menopause? She had many symptoms related to the condition.

Klara's husband was not entirely wrong. Many of our problems, including falls and loss of balance, can be related to the changing hormonal levels during menopause and after.

During our sexual cycles, most of us view menopause with ambivalence. We believe it will be a time free from any more hassles related to having periods, both physical and, to some extent, financial. But, when the time comes, we find ourselves struggling with mental and physical symptoms of menopause. What is more agonizing is the prolonged duration of this period. Menopause is not just a point or a pit stop. It is a *process* when our body and mind experience and endure complex involution changes.

The process, described as "normal" by medical textbooks, is a phase of our reproductive life cycle, commencing from age 45 to 55. This is the time when periods become irregular before they finally stop.

Menopause is associated with significant changes in sex hormone levels like estrogen and progesterone. Diminished estrogen secretion from the ovaries decreases its response to signals of brain hormones called follicle-stimulating hormone (FSH) and Luteinizing hormone (LH), further reducing estrogen secretion and actions in a negative feedback cycle.

When we progress toward menopause, these alterations in hormone levels cause symptoms. We increasingly have breakthrough bleeds that are not actual periods. Rising LH levels can cause red flushes, producing a burning skin sensation called "hot flushes."

An increasing vaginal and urinary dryness, associated with a decrease in estrogen levels, seems to be a bigger bother to many. It makes us more prone to urinary infections and pain during sexual intercourse. Reduced estrogen levels also increase the possibility of dysregulation of blood cholesterol levels, ischemic heart conditions, and high blood pressure.

Bone mass and density decrease due to the lowering of osteoclasts, the bone-modulating cells, actions. Estrogen plays a vital role in the growth and maturation of bone and in regulating bone turnover in adult bone. A fall in estrogen levels makes the bones weaker.

With many other things, we face the challenges of loss of balance.

Balance is a complex mechanism and requires integrated actions of various body processes. Proprioception, also known as kinesthesia, is the body's ability to sense its movement, activities, and position. It rests on gathering information from the surroundings through nerve receptors called proprioceptive receptors. These receptors are present in structures involved with movement and posture and include skin, bones, and muscles. The inputs gathered are called proprioceptive inputs.

Other sense organs pitch in. Our eyes help us to orient ourselves in our environment. So do the inner ears. The inner ears harbor sensitive hearing and proprioceptive organs called the vestibular system. These canals, sacs, and cavities are lined with sensitive hair-like structures and special cells that pick up information regarding our head position, spatial arrangement, and motion. The structural arrangement is small, approximately the size of a quarter, but they have crucial roles in maintaining balance with respect to our surroundings.

The data relating to these three conditions are continually transferred to the higher brain regions. The brain analyzes these data and relates them back to the organs of locomotion, bones, joints, and muscles to orient ourselves correctly in space. Thus, we can stand erect, walk tall, perform intricate body movements, and mold our bodies according to environmental requirements.

Balance also depends on strength and flexibility. We need these elements to keep our bodies upright and control their movements. Balance requires strong feet, legs, hips, bellies, and trunk muscles.

Aging affects our entire body systems. But we cannot allow it to touch our minds as well.

Accidents like the ones Klara and Anna had put us in perspective. We must do something to improve our balance to prevent sudden falls.

Research shows that balance declines in the middle years of life, commencing around 50. A study revealed that adults aged 30 years - 40 years could stand on one leg for a minute or more, which decreases to 45 seconds at 50 and 28 seconds at 70 years. The 80-year-olds could manage to stand on one leg for around 12 seconds (Balance begins to decline as early as age 50, 2022). The study also showed that 1/3rd of adults aged 56 years and more have one fall per year on average. While falls can be injurious to the body, they also break the mind.

To prevent and reduce the occurrence of falls in our golden years, we must become more aware of our bodies and their positions regarding our environment. We must exercise regularly to make our bones and muscles healthy and strong.

That is the only way to sustain our freedom.

I have trained students on the art and science of yoga for a considerable time to know and also to learn how yoga helps in regaining the strength and vitality of our bodies. While it rejuvenates the minds, the beauty of yoga is to root us in the space we belong, here and now.

We get back to strength, balance, and confidence.

The book on improving strength, balance, and preventing falls helps you to reduce the risk of falls, improve step length, and regain the confidence to walk without fear of falling. Consequently, you can prevent further injuries. You are able to overcome your general weakness and undertake your day-to-day activities safely.

The book has five chapters. Chapter One discusses how the body maintains its balance. It also tells us how internal weaknesses that we are unaware of can cause falls.

Chapter Two discusses the methods we can adopt to prevent falls. It includes refurbishing your home surroundings, using props, and guidance on proper footwear.

Chapter Three is on exercises to improve balance and stamina. It highlights the principles of yoga in enhancing our strength and toughness, including seated and standing poses focusing on strengthening the lower body, finding balance, and OTAGO Exercise programs.

Chapters Four and Five are on the yoga postures themselves. Follow the simple methods used to describe the asanas and do them to stay focused and balanced.

Chapter One

Bone Health & Balance

The balance of our body, sometimes considered our "sixth sense," depends on the health of the inner ear's vestibular system— the delicate canals and sacs with sense organs processing spatial information and information of our body's position and transferring them to the brain.

But it is not alone in its crucial task. The brain engages other organs to receive input, such as the eyes, the muscles, and the joints of our legs and back. But balancing our body erect, and maneuvering it, maintaining the equilibrium of both sides of the body in tandem mainly rests on the vestibular system.

In this regard, our ears perform unique functions. The rest of the sense organs, like the eyes, nose, and tongue, receive data on one thing only. For instance, the eyes can only see, the tongue taste, and the nose smell. But the ears, besides hearing, are also the balancing organs of the body. When we talk about ears, we are not referring to the fleshy outer structures we have on either side of our heads. The organ for balance lies deep within the bones of the skull and belongs to the inner ear.

But how does balance happen?

The Vestibular System of the Inner Ear

Balance

The vestibular system receives *information* from the five balance organs of the inner ear: the utricles, saccules, and the semicircular canals, eyes, muscles, and joints of the back and legs. The brain organizes the information and gives order to the different parts of the body to help maintain balance. Of all the sense organs, we rely primarily on our eyes to inform us of our spatial position.

The data sent by the inner ear sense organs involves the position of your head and orientation—the inner ear senses forward and backward, up and down, and circular motions. The sensory receptors vibrate at different frequencies of activity. While the inner ear responds best to relatively low-frequency movements, the eyes function best with higher-frequency motions.

The Brain

The brain learns about our position relative to our upright state and whether any motion is taking place. We allow the brain to correct our posture depending on the information we get. After the eyes, the inner ears are the second most important sense organ to send cues on position and posture to the brain; this is followed by the sensory nerves. In the absence of visual input, the other systems take over. Thus, if you try to maintain balance by closing your eyes, you rely on your inner ears and sensory nerves of the joints, muscles, and skin.

Karla, the doctors found, was suffering from sensorineural deafness that involved her balance organs. The doctors advised her to use ear aids and safe exercise methods.

Coming back to balance organs, the brain, in its turn, determines three modes of stability, eye, gait, and spatial orientation.

Eye or gaze stability: It coordinates eye and head movements. The visual system sends images of the environment surrounding us to the brain. If your eyesight is poor, you can have problems with balance.

Gait stability keeps us erect and stable on the ground, irrespective of the surface we are moving on.

Spatial stability maintains our body's equilibrium so that we do not topple over when we move.

Ensuring gaze stability: if you gaze fixedly at a point in front of you as you move your head from side to side, you will notice that instead of moving with your head, your eyes rotate to hold the gaze. It is the vestibular system that helps in the rotation of the eyes and is a reflex action.

Providing gait stability: To remain erect on one or both legs requires to-and-fro data sharing between the sensory organs or the proprioceptors of the bones, joints, leg and back muscles, and the brain. The sensory nerves in these areas respond to muscle tension due to posture, joint position, and pressures on areas of the soles of the feet. The brain resends back its directions after processing the data it receives. If you change your posture to walking or running, a new set of commands fired by the brain will keep you grounded.

Orienting in space (environment): Imagine a ride in the merry-go-round. The vestibular system helps you remain balanced in the whirlpool of movements you have subjected your body to. Similarly, when riding a car, an airplane, or a boat, there is a mismatch of motions between your body and your location. The vestibular system prevents you from falling in these situations.

When the vestibular system is functioning poorly, you can experience a loss of balance, falls, and dizziness.

Thus, balance keeps us erect, even when our external environment is rough or mobile. It helps us with normal gait, such as walking, jogging, running, or sprinting. We can move forward, backward, and sideways without falling down.

However, the system has its challenges. If you look at image projections on a large screen extending from ceiling to floor and both side walls, the images completely take up your visual fields, producing an illusion that you are within the environment.

You get an impression of being transported in an imaginary world instead of a spectator in a theater. You may move back and forth in your seat, mimicking a boat ride projected on the screen.

The information received from the eyes is processed in the motor cortex of the brain to enhance the precision of steps. We know where we are stepping, whether high or low, rough or even. When we encounter a block, for instance, a pothole or gravel, we make adjustments in motion to bypass it. The eyes help again by assessing the size and position of the obstacle.

The other brain region concerned with motion and balance is the cerebellum. It regulates gait through "error or correction" by responding to faulty postures for the corresponding environment. It senses the appropriate stepping patterns and compares them with the patterns you intend to make, correcting them accordingly. It sends more information to the brainstem and the motor cortex. Brainstem responses are instant corrections without making conscious choices.

Spinal reflexes maintain the rhythm of movement and gait stability. An example of a spinal stretch reflex in posture correction is leaning on one side from an erect posture. The corresponding back muscles of the other side begin to stretch; the sensory receptors in these muscle groups sense the stretch, and fire orders for them to contract. You regain your upright stance.

Strength of Body

Strong muscles, bones, ligaments, and healthy joints prevent falls and maintain proper gait and posture.

Muscle Tissues

Muscles can be of three types, skeletal, smooth, and cardiac. Of these, the skeletal muscles help with gait and locomotion. They are attached to bones by tendons. The other name for skeletal muscles is voluntary since the brain controls them.

Groups of muscles with opposing actions are attached around the joints. Thus, biceps muscles flexing the elbows are present in the front of the forearm. The triceps muscles at the back of the forearm oppose its actions by extending the forearm. Such an arrangement of muscles gives smooth motion and prevents injuries to any particular muscle group from overuse.

You can increase the size and strength of the skeletal muscles through regular exercise. Conversely, your muscles may weaken if you do not exercise for a long time.

Bones

Bones are constantly evolving structures. They give shape to our form and protection to the internal organs. The bones store calcium and phosphorus and produce the blood cells.

Bones grow in length during childhood, after which it increases in thickness. However, due to constant use, bone tissues undergo wear and tear. The body detects any weak spots and removes them by engaging bone cells called osteoclasts. New bone tissues replace these by the action of bone-forming cells. Hormone actions regulate the entire process, and estrogen plays a significant role. Minerals like calcium and vitamins like Vitamin D are essential for healthy bone formation. Bone formation is hampered by excessive smoking and drinking.

Bone formation declines steadily after 30 years. Regular exercise, particularly weight-bearing exercises, helps bone remodeling.

Changes With Aging

Movements take place in the joints. The interior of these structures is bathed in a protective and nourishing fluid called the synovial fluid. The amount of synovial fluid decreases with aging.

The bone ends forming the joints are covered by cartilage. Cartilage undergoes attrition with overuse and aging. The components of the cartilage, like the proteoglycans, also change, decreasing joint resilience. The joint surfaces do not slide as easily as they used to and is called osteoarthritis. The joint tissue becomes stiff, and the connective tissues get weaker and more brittle, affecting the range of joint motions.

Loss of muscle tissue or sarcopenia starts around 30 years and, like bone tissues, continues declining with aging. Muscle number, size, and amount are all reduced. Thus, there is a gradual loss of muscle mass and strength. Muscles that contract faster deteriorate more than those with slower contraction. You increasingly discover that things are falling from your hands, and your grip is no longer firm. Muscles cannot contract as quickly as they used to. As much as 50% of muscles can be lost by age 80. Muscles comprise 60% of our body mass, and significant loss of muscle mass can profoundly affect our health and well-being. The consequences of losing muscle tissue increase with aging, causing excessive weakness, higher incidence of falls, and loss of functionality and independence. Sarcopenia is associated with fatigue, insulin resistance, and rheumatological conditions (Walston, 2014).

Summary

The vestibular system of the inner ears maintains balance.

The sensory receptors in the eyes, ears, and connective tissues send cues or signals to the brain and spinal cord about our body in relation to spatial arrangement.

- Muscles and bones give strength.

- We lose muscles and bones with aging.
- Exercise prevents muscle and bone loss.
- The next chapter discusses methods to improve balance and strength.

Chapter Two

Methods to Improve Balance and Body Strength

It is one thing to think about doing something to build your body's strength and stamina and another to start dedicated programs to that effect. Any targeted action needs planning, organization, and execution. In this chapter, we will discuss how we can proceed to care for our health.

Health is equity, meaning we all deserve the highest standard of health. Regardless of gender, age, race, or social position, we all have the same fair opportunity to obtain optimum health and enjoy well-being.

Much as it sounds like jargon, optimal health ensures a balance between physical, emotional, social, spiritual, and intellectual balance, embracing a healthy lifestyle conducive to well-adjusted living. At the end of the day, we must feel satisfied with our efforts and achievements and have a restful night.

In other words, we come back to the WHO definition of health as physical, mental, and spiritual health, not just a lack of disease, condition, or weakness.

The key note here is to take things slowly but consistently.

For instance, if you are given to spending your days inactively, your body may be deconditioned to do any strenuous exercise. Sprinting to care for your leg and back muscles will injure them more.

Deconditioning is a medical term, meaning your body is unsuitable for endurance activities. It can happen after hospitalization, illnesses, or living an inactive lifestyle. There can be muscle weakness, stiffness of joints, restricted body movements, difficulties in standing for a longer time or performing daily activities without feeling too exhausted.

With aging, our coordination, decision-making, and mental acumen become slower, making adjustments challenging to introduce or follow. Nevertheless, once we start, we become more enthusiastic about ushering in lifestyle changes. Our effort's purpose is to become responsible for our health, or health self-advocacy.

Starting an exercise program is a journey requiring a step-by-step approach. We can use these five stages described in the transtheoretical model: pre-contemplation, contemplation, preparation, action, and maintenance.

The Five-Stage Model of Change

In the **pro-contemplation** stage, we are not seriously thinking about changing our lifestyle and refuse or ignore suggestions for help, including gathering health information. We continue to be defensive about our age-old habits, trying to justify them and why changing them would be difficult. We do not see any problem with our current way of living. We resist others' attempts to pressure us into making changes they believe are good for us.

The motivation or **contemplation** stage can happen anytime, even by reading this book. The fact that you are reading it shows your motivation for change. Why did you pick up the book? You may have been curious about strength training and a bit scared about losing muscle mass. Your increasing weakness and fatigue may have motivated you to seek ways to improve your health. Sometimes even a fall or an accident can trigger you to ask yourself why you lose balance and gait. You talk to your friends and doctors and read information on balance and body strength. You also contemplate your goals and what you desire out of a program. All our needs are unique, and your target areas may differ.

During this stage, you identify the roadblocks you may have and plan ways to overcome them. For instance, you feel unstable and wonder which exercise would not destabilize you. Our first aim in restoring health is not to do any harm. This Hippocratic oath abides in all healthcare segments, and yoga is no exception.

Yoga is an active, living science that you can modify to suit all ages, genders, and needs. Chair yoga is an excellent choice for you if you feel unstable on your foot in the beginning. You can move on to more vigorous exercises once you regain your stamina.

The next step after contemplation is the **preparation** for the journey to gain health. The milestones along the way depend upon the goals you set for yourself in the previous stage. If your motivation is building strength, you chalk out strength training programs; if you want to regain balance, you seek exercises that lean more on balance and posture but simultaneously focus on gradually increasing strength. You choose where you would like to exercise, the time, and any companion you would like to engage with in sharing your mission. You select the exercise programs most suitable for you at present. You find out what tools or gadgets you may require for the training. For example, you assess the necessity of joining a gym or choose the comfort of your home setting for a more relaxed program.

It may be helpful to journal your targets, exercise methods, plans regarding your diet, and rest time. Allot specific days for strength training and other days for different sets of exercises.

The next stage of this method is **action**. You start doing the exercises, a few to start with, and adjusting your coordination with the program before accelerating your efforts. You can appreciate the results of the changes you made. You feel stronger, better, and more content.

Theoretically, the action stage continues as long as you exercise. But after a period of six months, you transition to the final stage of **maintenance**. You have achieved your targets, like losing weight, feeling stronger, or more stable, and continue the endeavor to maintain the goodness achieved.

This is the time when strength and balance training become a part of your life. You do them out of practice, a routine that must be done to keep you energized throughout the day. Your body and mind act synergistically as if on a cue, propelled by an internal desire to exercise to stay fit.

You top up the effects by persisting with the other changes you made in your lifestyle, like good nutrition, adequate sleep, cultivating hobbies, and engaging in positive social interactions.

Requirements for Strength-Training

Strength training may not need any special instruments or gadgets; you can use your body to build strength. Indeed, walking itself is a good strength training program. Carry two water-filled one-liter bottles in your hands while you walk, and you can actually enhance your muscle strength. Other methods like pushups, planks, lunges, and squats all improve body strength and endurance.

Instruments that you can buy are resistance tubings. These are lightweight and inexpensive rubber tunes that give resistance. You wrap them around your body parts like the feet and pull the loose ends to feel the stretch, improving your core strength and balance. You can use them as props to perform various asanas with ease. They are available online, or you can buy them from a sports store.

Free weights, barbells, and dumbbells are typical tools for strength training. You can also use heavy books or water-filled bottles instead of using free weights. When you are using weights, start with smaller loads. For example, remove the load from one side of the dumbbells to reduce weight. Too much stress can injure weak muscles, and it is always better to start small and build up gradually.

Weight machines are an accessory to exercise programs. You must check your weight regularly to ensure any sudden loss or gain in weight.

Cable suspensions help you swing your body from a height, your feet lifted from the ground. This method of training that allows the body to work against gravity helps to build muscle and bone strength.

Balance Training

We need body balance for everything we do, from getting out of bed to tying our shoelaces. Balance requires the coordination of sense organs and the brain, but it also depends on the strength of your muscles and bones.

Balance training prevents falls and injuries. Balance training doesn't require many gadgets, and you can do them at home. The idea is to increase the strength and position sense of the muscles and joints that hold you upright. So your focus must be on the core, back, and leg muscles. Develop eye coordination with neck movements.

The exercises can be intensely active, like yoga. It draws your full attention to the body posture. Attention helps you understand your body's weak areas and how you should address them. It not only means improving your weaknesses but also thinking about methods that can reduce falls.

Simple balance exercises can involve standing on a leg for a few seconds.

A Bosu half-circle stability ball or a balance board are some gadgets that offer you balance training programs.

Accessories

Home settings for exercise training must be safe and secure. If you decide to join a gym, try to locate a facility catering to women of your age group. Let them know about any health conditions you might have. Ask for a guided tour of the facility to ensure proper lighting, space, cleanliness, and staff behavior.

Homes can be remodeled for moving around and exercise without much effort. Get the full benefits from the programs by adhering to the following rules.

Choose the designated area for exercise. Use this space and no other whenever you are exercising.

Move away all the furniture. Spread a soft rug on the floor. It must not have frayed edges, loose ends, or holes. Alternatively, use a yoga mat.

Ensure proper lighting and heating. Arrange the temperature setting according to your preference. You may need cooler temperatures while you exercise.

Use a chair for seated chair yoga. Additionally, you may need a low bench for bench press. Select a stable chair without armrests.

If you are prone to falls, use safety methods like an alarm system that you can wear as a bracelet. Pushing a button if you fall while exercising will alert emergency medical personnel. Take your time receiving the call. Install an answering machine, carry a cordless one, or keep your cell phone handy during training.

Exercise is a training program with specific needs. Acknowledging them would be best. Besides a safe environment and tools, you need suitable **footwear** to support your body during the exercise. You cannot do them wearing flip-flops. You will not be able to do the full range of motions wearing fancy or flimsy shoes or trying to do the asanas barefoot. Furthermore, you may injure your bones and ligaments. Throughout the training, you must support the arch of your feet by wearing good-quality orthopedic or athletic shoes. Use lightweight slip ons of elastic fabric, which are rubber-soled and without heels. They grip the yoga mat and support you while you execute the asanas.

Nutrition

Appetite tends to decrease with aging. We often skip meals. We drink less water, increasing dehydration. Exercise, especially yoga asanas, improves appetite in several ways.

Eat breakfast properly; your lunch must be moderately heavy and your dinner light.

Eat three meals and two snacks between meals.

Avoid junk foods and oily foods. Eat seasonal and fresh foods. Include plenty of green vegetables, legumes, and fruits of all colors in your diet.

Eat whole grain cereals.

Eat a handful of nuts, dried fruits, and seeds or fruit for snacking.

Reduce red meat and alcohol.

Eat poultry and fish at least two to three times a week.

Have yogurt, and drink low-fat milk. If you are allergic to milk, use soy milk or almond milk instead.

Drink plain water frequently and with meals.

Use Vitamin D supplementation and calcium tablets.

Other Lifestyle Choices

Avoid smoking.

Engage in meaningful and positive social interactions. Aim at building relationships.

Engage in hobbies that you love. Gardening, nature walking, sewing, and painting can all be beneficial for improving your mood and attention.

Learn a new skill or knowledge.

Sleep at least seven to eight hours at night.

Take a day off to be on your own. You can watch a movie, eat out, or visit a friend. A day spent differently will re-establish your routine with a sense of purpose.

Practice meditation to improve mindfulness and concentration.

Medical Check-Ups

Check your blood pressure and blood sugar levels. If you are already on any medications, ask your doctor if you need any adjustments of timings with the exercises.

Check your eyesight and ears for visual and hearing acuity.

If you have a family history of osteoporosis or one of your parents had a fractured hip or back, get a DXA scan to rule out osteoporosis.

Summary

- Do exercises regularly.
- Do strength training exercises 2 - 3 times weekly.
- Eat nutritious foods and drink water.
- Avoid smoking and reduce alcohol use.
- Engage in positive hobbies.

The next chapter is on specific exercises to improve balance and stamina. It highlights the principles of yoga in enhancing our strength and endurance.

Chapter Three

Exercises to Improve Balance & Prevent Falls

All adults require at least 150 minutes of moderate-intensity exercise every week. Spread it over at least five days a week. Any activity that raises your heart rate by 50% - 60% from normal is moderate intensity. You can talk, but you cannot sing during moderate-intensity training. However, if it is impossible to do this level of exercise, do what you can comfortably. Any activity is better than none at all. Some examples of moderate-intensity exercise are as follows:

- Walking two miles in 30 minutes.
- Swimming for 20 minutes.
- Dancing for 30 minutes.
- Water aerobics for 30 minutes.
- Washing a car for 45 minutes.
- Gardening for 30 to 45 minutes.
- Pulsing a lawn mower.

Exercises for Strength

Perform **Strength training** for all major muscle groups at least twice a week. A 20-minute session on each of these occasions is sufficient to bring a noticeable improvement in your strength. A **single set** of each exercise, with a weight or resistance band for 12 to 15 repetitions, or until you tire the muscles, is considered adequate (Androulakis-Korakakis, 2020). With time, lifting more weights for a longer duration will be possible. This is when your muscle mass is actually increasing, and bone strength is gaining. Some examples of strength training are as follows:

- Lifting weights
- Dancing

- Groceries carrying
- Climbing up and down the stairs
- Aerobics to music
- Heavy gardening work, such as digging or shoveling
- Yoga

Exercises for Balance & Flexibility

Activities to improve balance and flexibility twice weekly reduce the risk of falling. Yoga is the best method to improve balance (Youkhana, 2016). It can reduce joint stiffness and improve unsteady gait.

Do not spend time sitting for a long time. Get up after every 20 - 30 minutes, take a stroll, and return to work.

Exercising with Osteoporosis

Osteoporosis increases the risk of fractures of the spine and hip. It is better to seek medical guidance before starting to exercise. While lifting weights, keep your knees bent. Avoid stooping low or lifting movements and high-impact exercises. Of all forms of exercise, yoga is beneficial in osteoporosis also.

Yoga for Strength & Balance

Yoga is a Hindu philosophy of *union* or *yoga* between the body, mind, and spirit. It is not a religion but a code to practice a healthy and well-balanced life. In that respect, yoga is practical and hence popular. The other reasons for its popularity are the ease of doing yoga anytime, anywhere, with very few resources. We can all do yoga, and numerous studies have shown that yoga improves balance and flexibility, reduces stiffness and joint pain, and improves core strength. The asana(s) are gentle body folds coordinated with breathing. You can smoothly flow from one asana to another without feeling tired. The benefits of yoga include the following:

- Boost energy
- Improve muscle tone and sculpt the body
- Better fine motor coordination
- Better flexibility
- Improved postural alignment
- Improved cardiovascular fitness
- Reduction of arthritis pain
- Improvement of digestive ailments
- Improvement of sleep
- Reduction of depression and anxiety
- Improved bone density in women over 50

OTAGO Exercise Programs

The New Zealand Falls Prevention Research Group in New Zealand designed the Otago Exercise Program (OEP) to reduce falls in older persons. Studies show OEP participants experience a 35% – 40% reduction in falls.

It comprises 17 strength and balance exercises and a walking program, thrice weekly by the seniors in their homes, outpatient, or community settings. Do them individually or as a group participant.

The program is most effective for frail seniors. After an evaluation by a physical therapist, you can do the prescribed exercises. Exercises are performed under the guidance of the physical therapist, PT Assistant, or an appropriate healthcare provider for 2 months. Transition to the self-management phase continues for 4 -10 months, with monthly monitoring over the phone and an optional 6 monthly visits to the center.

Doing the Asanas

Clear any clutter from the area where you will exercise regularly. It can be objects like toys for your grandchildren, pet toys, small rugs, furniture, electrical wires, wi-fi lines, electrical extension cords, books, and any other things that you can suddenly step on and trip.

Avoid glaring lights, distractions from television noises, darkness, and hot, humid temperatures.

Wear cotton or breathable outfits, loose and comfortable but not overflowing.

Wear good shoes with socks.

Keep a water bottle handy and stay hydrated.

Remain aware of your body position and stance throughout the exercise. Pay attention to sore spots. It is normal to develop mild soreness over the body after beginning your program, but these disappear after a few days of rest. However, if the pain persists and is sharp, consult your doctor.

Do what you can tolerate. Push yourself a little at a time. For instance, you might try holding an asana for five seconds longer.

Allow a day off for recovery. On these days, you may substitute routine exercise with other methods like gardening or mindful walking in nature.

Before commencing, do a few warm-up asanas. It should last for five minutes. Warm-ups gradually increase blood flow to the muscles and joints and build up heart rates. Joint flexibility and muscle temperatures increase. You can enjoy a better range of movements with the actual asanas.

End the asanas with cooldowns. Your muscles come back to their resting state, heart rate and breathing slow down, and your body bursts into cooling sweat. It prevents muscle fatigue. You also become aware of developing any injury at this time.

Many online video content can show the wrong techniques, and as a result, you may injure yourself or practice asanas without getting benefits. Verify the authenticity of the videos you follow.

Ensure all your equipment is safe.

You may summon someone to watch while doing the asanas for safety's sake. They can check that you are doing the asanas correctly and also ensure your safety. Once you mold into the practice, you can do them alone.

Summary

Seniors must do at least 150 minutes weekly of moderate-intensity exercise.

Split it over at least five days a week.

Combine it with twice-weekly single-set strength training for 20 - 30 minutes.

Yoga is one of the best exercises to build bone density and balance in women over 50.

The next two chapters discuss the different asanas.

Chapter Four
Asanas to Improve Strength

Falls are undoubtedly inconvenient. Besides exposing our weaknesses and diminishing body control, sometimes embarrassingly, they are injurious to limbs, back, and sometimes to the brain, causing a concussion. The incidence of falls increases with age above 65 years.

The muscles that prevent falls are the core, leg, and upper limb muscles. We will focus on each of these parts and describe asanas to improve their strength.

The Core Muscles

The core, or the trunk of the body, comprises a group of 29 muscles and forms the body's foundation. It includes the diaphragm, pelvic floor, spine, hips, and abdominal muscles. Our core stabilizes hip and shoulder girdles and protects the spine from injuries. A weak core makes us feel less steady on our feet, and we find trouble getting out of a chair or a car. We can perform weight-bearing activities like lifting grocery bags or climbing stairs. We can participate in sports activities like tennis and golf.

To work the core, we must do asanas involving the hip, lower back, and abdominal muscles.

Improve your core strength with yoga by doing the following exercises.

Core-strengthening Asanas

Most core-strengthening exercises require coordination and action of multiple muscle groups and are best down at the ground level. However, if getting down is challenging, use a chair or a cushioned wide bench that supports your body weight while doing the asana.

Be kind to your body as you do the asanas. Hold on to support whenever necessary. Relax between repetitions and after an asana. Do not worry if you falter.

Warm-Up

Start yoga with warm-ups like marching on the spot.

Method

- Stand tall on a mat in a tadasana pose. Your gaze should be forward, hands by your sides, shoulders rolled back, legs straight with toes pointing forward, and the knees locked.
- Place the heel of the right foot in front of the left, letting it touch the toes of the feet behind.
- Maintain your stance, and gaze forward.
- Now, step the left foot forward, simultaneously taking the right foot back. Try to hold your balance.
- If it is challenging to do this pose standing, use a stable chair.
- Repeat the back-and-forth on-spot marching movements to warm up the leg muscles.

Other warm-ups can include easy sways from side to side or making gentle kicks in the air. Your hands can be at your sides or move in rhythm with the body.

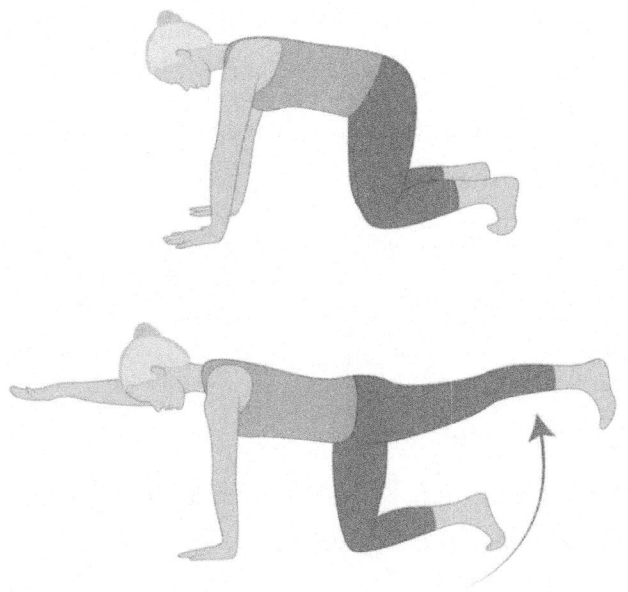

Bird Dog

Method

- Use a cushioned wide bench to do the pose if getting down on floor level is challenging. Hold each movement for a few seconds before moving on to the next stage. Inhale during making the movements and exhale when you come back to rest. Breathe evenly in between.
- Keep your back straight and your hips aligned with your trunk. For pain in the wrist or ankle joints, use an exercise ball to lie on it and do the asana. It will remove pressure on these joints.
- Kneel on all fours on a mat. Keep your knees at hip-width apart. Your arms must be directly below the shoulders.
- Inhale and tighten your abdomen by squeezing the belly button. Your neck and shoulders must be relaxed.

- Move your right arm straight in front of you, your thumb pointing upward.
- Raise your arm as high as possible but not above your ear.
- Try raising the left leg behind you, holding it straight in the air.
- Hold the pose for a few breaths.
- Exhale and lower your right arm. Then, lower the left leg.
- Repeat the asana on the other side.

Hold on to a chair seat for support if this pose is challenging.

Easy Bird Dog

Method

- Kneel on all fours on the bench. Keep your knees at hip-width apart. Your arms must be directly below the shoulders.
- Inhale and tighten your abdomen by squeezing the belly button. Your neck and shoulders must be relaxed.
- Keep your right arm straight, your thumb pointing upward.
- Raise your arm as high as possible but not above your ear.
- Lower the right arm on the mat upon exhalation.
- Repeat the asana with the left arm.
- Then, raise the right leg behind your back and hold it straight, toes pointing downward.
- Exhale and lower the leg.
- Repeat the motion on the left side.

Knee Plank

Plank is a complete workout that strengthens the core, legs, arms, and shoulders.

Do not feel daunted by the pose; you can always start it by doing a simpler knee plank and then moving on to a full-body plank when you gain more strength and balance.

Method

- Lie on your face on the cushioned bench that can support your weight.
- Bend your forearms at the elbows, keeping them close to your chest and the thumbs pointing up.
- Lift up your body at the hips; your knees should remain on the ground.
- Now, lift the heels straight in the air, both legs joining each other.
- Your body rests on the forearms and at the hips.
- Hold your back and your hips in one straight line. Lift your heels at this height.
- Hold this posture for 60 seconds or as long as you can.

Full Plank

Method

- Lie on a mat on your face.
- Bend the forearms at the elbows, keeping them near the chest.
- Inhale and lift up your whole body, your legs resting only on the toes.
- Your body should form one straight line from head to toe.
- Hold the position for 12 - 15 seconds and release.
- Repeat the asana to make a total of 60 seconds.

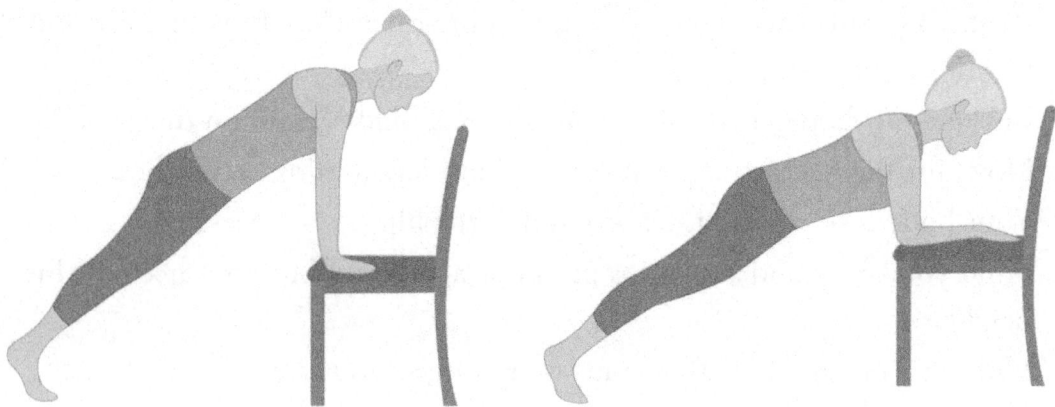

Chair Plank Pose

It can be challenging for you to lie down on the floor. Still, you can do the plank using a kitchen chair. Avoid using too small chairs with wide seats.

Method

- Take a stable chair without armrests.
- Bend forward on the chair, firmly holding its sides. Your shoulders should be right above the palms.
- Step back, supporting your foot on the heels.
- Your neck, back, hips, and shoulders should form a straight line.
- Tighten the core and the hips.
- Relax.
- You can do gentle push ups in this posture.

Alternative Chair Plank

Method

- Sit tall on a backless chair.
- Extend your hands and legs forward. Rest your feet on the heels. Keep your hips in the center, and sit on your tailbone.
- Now roll back your shoulders as you gradually lean backward, your neck, shoulders, and back forming a straight line.
- Hold the position for 30 seconds and come back to rest.

Side Plank Pose

The side plank works the side abdominals, rib, leg, and arm muscles. You can do the asana lying on a mat or using a cushioned wide bench if getting down on the floor is difficult.

Method

- Lie on your right side on a wide bench.
- Bend the right arm, keeping the forearm on the ground.
- Bend the knees forward at 45° with the ankles.
- Lift the hips from the ground using your fist. With more practice, you can do this step without using the fist as support.
- Hold your body in a straight line.
- Place the left arm on your body and hold the position as long as you can or for a minute.
- Repeat on the left side.
- Once you gain strength, keep your legs straight instead of folding them at the knees. Your weight will be on the forearm and the ankles.
- Repeat on the other side.

Upward-Facing Knee Bent Pose

Also called *urdhamukha janusirasana* in Sanskrit, this asana is a modification of the janu sirsasana. It is a version of the Palloff press and works wonders on all strengthening muscle groups of the body.

Method

- You can sit on a chair and use another chair or a bench to lift up your leg. Alternatively, you can sit on a mat. You will need a resistance band to do the exercise.
- Sit tall on a chair.
- Lift up your right knee on the seat, and let your foot rest against the inner thigh of the left leg.
- Loop the resistance bend around your left heel and hold the ends in both hands.
- Straighten your back and stretch both arms, pulling the band toward you.
- Tilt your head back and breathe slowly in and out.
- Hold the pose for 30 seconds.
- Release.
- Repeat on the other side.

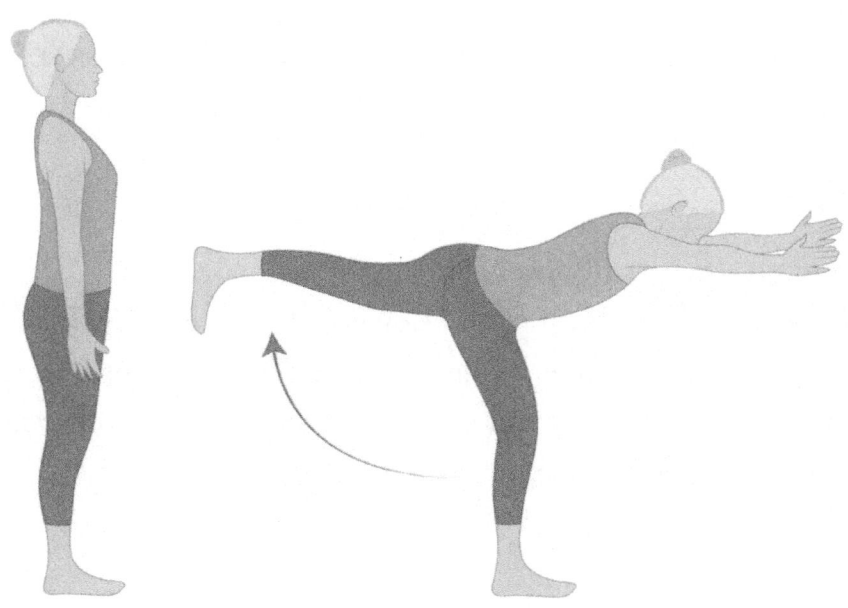

Standing Superman Pose

In Sanskrit, this asana is called *viparita salabhasana*. You can do it standing.

Method

- Stand tall on a mat.
- Lift your left knee behind you, your foot facing the ground.
- Raise both arms straight toward the ceiling.
- Now, slowly tilt forward, bringing your arms down, until both your arms are facing forward.
- Your whole body now rests on your right leg.
- Hold the position for 20 - 30 seconds.
- Relax and repeat on the other side.

Hold on to a chair seat for support if this pose is challenging. As you gain more strength, try to release the support gradually.

Leg lifts

Also called *utthita hasta padangusthasana* in Sanskrit, do this asana standing or seated in a chair.

Method

- Stand on a mat or sit on a chair.
- Tighten your belly button, and slowly lift your right leg 5″ off the floor.
- Stand tall, your shoulders rolled back, and hold the position for 30 seconds.
- Lower it on the ground and repeat the exercise on the other side.
- Do this exercise 10 times on each side.

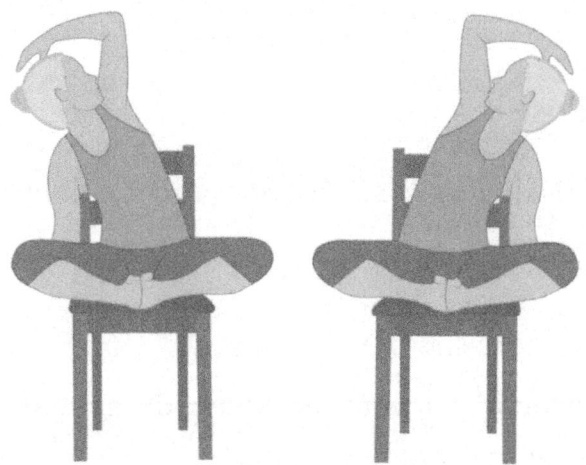

Seated Side Bend Pose

Method

- Sit tall on a chair with no arms, like a kitchen chair or an exercise ball.

- Place your right hand behind your head.
- Extend your left arm down towards the floor.
- Inhale and tighten the right side of your abdomen, and face right as you lean over to the right and come back to the center. Keep your back straight and remain sitting on your tailbone.
- Now, raise the left arm behind your head. Your right arm should be beside you.
- Turn left and contract the left side of your abdomen.
- Repeat the asana 5 - 10 times on each side.
- Do this 10 times on the right side and repeat on the left.

Seated Clam-shell Pose

Method

Sit tall on a chair, your legs at hip-width apart and your feet firmly on the ground.

- Your knees should be above the ankles.
- Wrap a resistance band around your shin bones.
- Now tighten the core and pull the band apart by separating your thighs. Keep your back straight, your hands resting on the side of the chair or your thighs.
- Hold the pose for 30 seconds and relax.

The Woodchopper Pose

The yoga pose strengthens the abdomen, and lower body, quickens the heart rate, and challenges your body. You can do the Woodchopper pose standing. In Sanskrit, it is called kastha-takshanasana.

Method

- Stand tall with your feet at hip-width apart. Gaze forward, your chin facing forward.

- Fold your legs at the knee to a squatting position.
- Inhale, clasping your hands together above your head, and as you forcefully exhale, bring them down between your thighs in one swift motion.
- Make 10 repetitions of this asana.

The Leg Muscle

Balance

Of all the leg muscles, it is essential to pay attention to the big muscles like the hamstrings and the quadriceps to maintain posture and balance. When they are strong, we can easily get up from a seated or lying position and walk correctly. The smaller muscles around the ankles and feet maintain balance and prevent bone fractures from minor injuries.

Mountain Pose With Head-Turning

This is a great pose to learn to balance your body while turning the head. In a real-life scenario, you have to do this to look at the traffic or talk to a friend while walking. You can also do the pose seated.

Method

- Stand tall, feet hip-width apart, and facing forward.
- Bring your palms toward your chest and interlock the fingers.
- Turn your palms inside out and exhale as you straighten your hands in front of you. Your fingers should stay interlocked. Hold the pose for 30 seconds.
- Now inhale, raise your hands above your head, and gradually turn your head toward the right side, back to center, and then left.
- Add zest to the pose by slowly marching forward and turning your head toward the sides. You can also hold your hands ahead while marching.

Sit-to-Stand Yoga Pose

Method

- Stand tall in a mountain pose facing a chair, your feet at hip-width.
- Bend your knees, raising both your hands upward in a chair pose until your bottom reaches the chair seat.
- Push yourself back to the standing pose without taking the support of the chair. Exert force through your heels.
- Repeat the move 10 times.

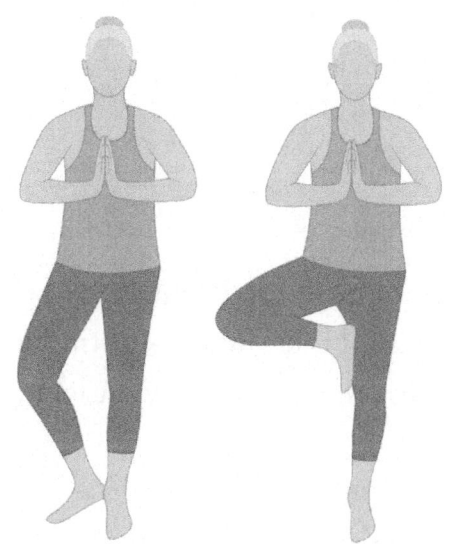

One-Legged Prayer Pose

It is one of the most valuable balance poses. Use a chair for support if necessary.

Method

- Stand tall with your feet hip-width apart.

- Slowly lift your right foot off the floor. You can hold the pose here or proceed to the next steps.
- Bring the right foot across to the left leg and rest it on the inner side of the left thigh. You can use your hands to adjust the leg in position.
- Keep your back straight as you bring your palms to your chest in a namaste or payer sign. Instead, hold the back of the chair if you want support.
- Hold the posture as long as you can.
- Release, relax, and repeat on the other side.

Cool-Down

Cool-down is as important as the warm-up.

Legs up the Wall Pose

Method

- Place a chair facing a wall.
- Sit sideways on your right side and bring your knees to your chest so your bottom touches the wall. Hold the sides of the chair for balance.
- Now turn toward your left and extend your legs on the wall. Your back can rest on the chair back.
- You can spread the legs in a V-shape.
- End the pose by folding your legs to your chest. Hold the sides of the chair as you roll to one side.

Summary

- Core strengthening is crucial to fall prevention.
- Strengthen the leg muscles to better balance.
- Do the asanas slowly and take time to adjust.

Chapter Five

Some More Asanas

To prevent falls, we must have a strong core. Additionally, a strong lower body part helps us maintain gait and balance. Similarly, upper body strength is crucial to many of our daily functions like gripping, holding, grasping, lifting, or catching. Even a simple chore like cleaning the house and mopping requires reliable upper-body coordination. This chapter will discuss upper-body strengthening exercises, more balance poses, and some OTEG exercises.

We will start with a warm-up which is balancing as well.

Lateral Step

Method

- Stand with your feet hip-width apart.
- Focus on a point on the wall. You can draw one on the wall or place a flyer.
- Begin to lean on the right until you can lean no further. Step to the right at this point.
- Come back to rest.
- Repeat it on the other side.
- Do it five times on both sides.

Asanas to Strengthen the Upper Body

Reverse Tabletop

This pose works wonders for the triceps and the shoulders, besides opening and stretching the chest. You would need a stable chair without an armrest.

Method

- Sit on a chair.
- Hold the sides of the chair.
- Keep your legs on the floor shoulder-width apart and your knees at 90° with the ankles.
- Inhale and lift the hips from the chair, raising your body from the chair seat. Your feet should be firm on the ground and squeeze the hip muscles.
- Hold the position for 30 seconds.
- Exhale and come back to the seated posture.
- Relax.

Bound Hands Humble Warrior Flow Pose

An intermediate vinyasa yoga, the bound hands humble warrior pose flow requires having your hands bound behind the body.

Method

- Stand tall in *tadasana*, palms facing forward.
- Keep your arms to the sides and open up your chest.
- Inhale and bring your left foot forward, and bend it at the knee just above the left ankle. Your right foot should be straight back; toes pointed inward.
- Exhale and take your arms behind your body, and as you inhale, clasp them behind you.
- Now breathe in and out as you lift your chest and neck.
- Gradually fold forward, raise your clasped hands toward the ceiling as you fold forward toward the left knee.
- Hold the pose for 5 - 8 breaths and relax.
- Repeat on the other side.

Standing Side Arm Raises

This asana helps to build muscle mass in the upper body.

Method

- Stand tall in *tadasana* and shift your weight to the right leg as you move the left leg sideways.
- Your feet should be firmly on the ground.
- Roll back and relax your shoulders.
- Lift both arms out at the sides and slightly bend them at the elbows. They must not be above shoulder height.
- Hold the position for 30 seconds.
- Relax.
- Do 5 repetitions.
- Go back to *tadasana*.
- Now shift your weight to the left leg and move your right leg sideways.
- Repeat the rest of the movements.
- Do 5 repetitions.
- As you develop strength, add hand weights to do the exercise.

Seated Lean with Weights

Doing this pose teaches you to control your core and bodyweight transference. You can do the exercise on a chair, a couch, or an exercise ball. The exercise ball can add an extra challenge to balance because of its sloping surface.

- Sit tall on a chair and hold the ends of a water-filled bottle or a weight in both hands.
- Bring the weight to your chest level.
- Raise your arms slowly above your head. Press on the weight all the time.

- Now, inhale and lean to your right, keeping your back straight. Appreciate the stretch at the left side of your body.
- Exhale as you come back to the center.
- Inhale and lean toward the left. And come back to center as you exhale.
- Repeat the movements on each side five times, flowing with your breath.

Asana to Enhance Balance

Heel Lifts

This yoga exercise enhances the balance and strength of the calf muscles.

- Sit tall on a chair with your feet on the floor and hip-width apart.
- Inhale, bend slightly forward, press on your toes, and start lifting yourself up on your toes. Move as high as possible and slowly lower the heels on the ground.
- You can hold a chair in front for support. Conversely, to add challenge, you can raise your hands in front of you.
- As you get accustomed, keep your spine straight when you lift yourself up.
- Repeat 10 times.

Goddess Pose

This asana strengthens and lengthens hips, groin, inner thighs, knees, ankles, and pelvic floor muscles.

Method

- Stand tall in *tadasana*.
- Inhale and spread your legs apart, toes pointing outward and heels inward. Take care to maintain your trunk neutral and even.
- Tighten your core, and as you exhale, squat, bending the knees. Your knees must not protrude beyond the ankles.

- After ensuring your lower body is balanced, open your arms at the sides with the next inhalation, keeping them bent at the elbows. Your palms must be open and face forward.
- Look ahead, roll back your shoulders, and breathe into the pose for 5 - 8 breaths.
- Exhale, bringing the arms by your side and straightening the knees.
- Come back to mountain pose.
- You can add variations to the goddess pose by raising alternate legs while lifting the arms at your sides. Stand tall for this variation instead of squatting.

Foot-to-Seat Pose

Method

- Stand in front of a chair.
- Place your hand on the back of the chair.
- Step the right foot on the chair seat.
- Raise the right hand toward the ceiling.
- Keep your back straight and gaze ahead.
- Hold the posture for 30 seconds and repeat on the other side.

Clock Reach Pose

You'll need a chair for this exercise.

- Stand tall behind a chair. Hold its back with your left hand.
- Lift your right leg, and move your right arm forward, holding it at an imaginary 12 o'clock position of a watch.
- Keeping your right leg raised, swipe your right arm sideways. Imagine you are moving your arm like the minute hand of a clock and pause briefly at each 5-minute position from 12 o'clock.
- Continue the rotation movement of the arm until you reach your back at an imaginary 6 o'clock position.

- From here, bring your arm back to the 12 o'clock position.
- Look ahead during the entire exercise.
- Repeat it on the other side.
- To add challenge, keep your left hand straight in front as you move the right hand sideways, and try to follow the right hand's movement.

Straddle Squats Side

- Stand in tadasana.
- Separate your feet to stand in a straddle position.
- Gaze ahead and lift the arms forward.
- Exhale, bringing the right knee, coming to a side squat.
- Lift the fingertips and switch to the other side.
- Inhale, come to the center and exhale side squat.
- Get as close to the ground as possible to do the squats.
- Take the support of your fingertips to help you do the deep squats as you sweep from side to side.
- Inhale as you come to the center and exhale as you do the side squats.

Otago Strengthening Exercises

Do these strengthening exercises guided by the OTAGO program. Do them thrice weekly, with one intervening rest day (Otago Exercise Program Activity Booklet, n.d.).

Front Knee Strengthening Exercise

Method

- Sit in a chair, resting your back against the chair back.
- Strap the weight onto your right ankle.
- Straighten the leg.
- Repeat 10 times.

- Strap the weight around the left ankle.
- Straighten the left leg, keeping the right leg on the ground.

Back Knee Strengthening Exercise

- Strap the weight on your right ankle.
- Stand up tall, and support yourself by holding the back of the chair.
- Bend the knee backward, and raise the foot toward your hips.
- Release.
- Repeat 10 times.
- Strap the weight on your left ankle.
- Repeat the exercise on your left side 10 times.

Side Hip Strengthening Exercise

Method

- Strap the weight on your right ankle.
- Stand up tall behind a chair and hold it.
- Keep your legs straight, your feet facing forward.
- Raise the right leg to the side and return to the neutral position.
- Repeat 10 times.

Calf Raises

- Stand up tall, facing a chair and holding it for support. Look ahead.
- Keep your feet shoulder-width apart.
- Lift yourself on your toes.
- Lower the heels to the floor.
- Repeat this exercise 10 times.
- As you gain strength, try doing the exercise without support.

Otago Balance Exercises

Enjoy doing these simple balancing activities every day.

Knee Bends

Method

- Stand tall, facing a chair and holding it for support.
- Keep your feet shoulder-width apart.
- Bend your knees and squat down halfway. Your knees should be over the toes. Stand up when your heels have started lifting from the floor.
- Repeat 10 times.
- Try to exercise without support when you gain more strength and balance.

Backward Walking

Method

- Stand up tall and hold the back of a table.
- Walk 10 steps backward, following the length of the table.
- Turn around and hold the table with your other hand.
- Walk backward 10 steps to the start point.
- Repeat 10 times.
- You can do this exercise without using the table's support.

Walking and Turning Around

Method

- Stand near a table.
- Start walking at an even pace.
- Make a clockwise turn.
- Walk back to the initial position.

- Now, turn counter-clockwise
- Move, making repetitions of the figure of eight movements.

Sideways Walking

Without Support

Method

- Stand up tall near a table and try walking without holding it.
- Take 10 steps to the left.
- Take 10 steps to the right.
- Repeat the activity

Heel Toe Walking

Method

- Stand up tall near a table and look forward.
- Place one foot directly in front of the other, your feet forming a straight line. Place the foot behind directly in front of the front foot.
- Repeat for 10 more steps.
- Turn around and repeat the movement.

Stair Walking

Method

- Hold the handrail of a staircase and slowly climb up, one step at a time.
- Turn round when you reach the next landing and climb down.

Conclusion

As we age, it is normal to lose body strength and flexibility. Body processes slow down and are not as efficient as before. The food we eat is not fully absorbed or metabolized; we feel less hungry and active. We feel lethargic and sluggish. Yet, we may not sleep well at night. Our eyesight weakens, and our hearing is not sharp. How often have our family members told us we do not listen to what they say? We may blame our faltering attention on hearing loss, but it is also true that we tend to lose our grip on the present moment. All of this and loss of joint sense and balance contribute to falls and accidents. They increase over time, becoming more frequent in the 80s.

While our lifespan increases, we must try to live it well. We may not be able to control our future, but we can take care of the present.

Yoga is the best therapeutic approach to all types of aging problems. The asanas restore the balance of the body, mind, and spirit. As you do the asanas, you understand how it is made possible by yoga. You realize that you must focus on your activities here and now, wanting to challenge you to do better and more. The exercises make you feel happy and satisfied. You can even add tweaks to enhance your skills.

Read the book, do the asanas, and enjoy your freedom to move indoors and outdoors without falling.

Mindful Chair Yoga

Lasting Relaxation for Seniors. Safe & Comfortable Sequences to Help Sleep Problems, Relieve Stress and Build Your Inner Calm

Introduction

At 57, Gloria was at the crossroads of her life. She had dedicated her prime to raising two children. Both were now grown-up adults ready to leave home. Gloria would have been all right with it had they decided to settle somewhere within the country. But both were going abroad, to lands Gloria knew nothing about. The uncertainty of the turn of events was stressful. The idea of loneliness and estrangement pervaded her nights and days.

Gloria found she could not concentrate on her daily tasks. She forgot essential things. Her family members and friends were increasingly noticing how absent-minded she had been lately. But Gloria would respond unequivocally to their concerns or complaints.

She was restless and agitated. Often, she would get up and pace the room, sometimes for hours, apparently lost in her thoughts.

When talking to others, she would fidget, pull her hair, or pick her skin.

Gloria's husband took her to the family doctor. He wanted her to have a health check. He was surprised when the doctor suggested a psychiatric evaluation for Gloria.

Doctors diagnosed Gloria with a generalized anxiety disorder or GAD. The doctor believed her "empty nest syndrome" feelings were possibly linked to menopause and age-related chronic ailments like high blood pressure and generalized weakness. One thing led to another and undermined Gloria's confidence. She lost belief in her abilities to withstand physical and emotional tensions and enjoy *her* life as best as possible, leading to stress and nervous agitation.

The doctor prescribed medications for Gloria. They also advised her to exercise regularly and practice mindfulness. She should manage her nutrition, sleep well, and make other healthy lifestyle changes.

Regarding exercises, the doctor suggested Gloria practice chair yoga, as she lacked endurance and mental flexibility for rigorous training. Yoga would be gentle on her body and mind and help her to sleep well at night. Simultaneously, she would learn to become more aware of herself and her immediate environment.

Through yoga, Gloria would understand the mutual dependency between her surroundings and herself and reflect on the support she had consistently received from the environment she knew. Her inward journey, aided by gentle chair yoga, will rekindle Gloria's trust in her abilities, her support systems, and the overall goodness of things. Most importantly, she would discover a new purpose and regain control over *her* life.

Truda was pushing 55, but unlike Gloria, she had been very busy with her professional life. But Truda, the enthusiastic CEO of a giant multinational, was lately feeling the strain of workplace load and home obligations. She was a compulsive worker, almost a workaholic who efficiently juggled home and work environments. However, she now found work uninteresting, a mere drudgery. Her professional life drained her energy and left her exhausted to pursue self-care routines, hobbies, or social activities. Truda's stress showed in her interactions with close family members. She was irritated, strained, and sometimes aggressive. Truda recognized her mood swings but didn't know why she had them. There were *no possible reasons* as far as her life was concerned. But she could not sleep at night. She stopped watching the television as a corrective measure and went to bed early. She listened to calming music to sleep better. But nothing helped. She woke up in the morning feeling depressed and tired.

Truda's worried family members suggested that she must seek medical advice.

Truda neglected it for a while until one day, she collapsed at work. Her colleagues rushed her to the emergency. Truda had a psychiatric evaluation, among other investigations. She was diagnosed with depression. The doctor prescribed medications and advised yoga as an exercise routine. Yoga could help Truda get more oriented toward her life goal and help her achieve it.

How can one method give you all you need to improve and maintain your physical, mental, and spiritual health? Increasingly, medical professionals believe in therapies like yoga to restore strength, endurance, and body flexibility. They acknowledge that yoga is also the best mindfulness technique.

The ancient Sanskrit-speaking philosophers and teachers designed yoga as a bridge between our inner selves and the higher power that governs the universe. We all belong to that force and draw our energy from it. However, our social background and traditional education insulate us from this intrinsic truth.

We rush through life events without focusing on the merits of the things we possess: our spirit and mind. We get more concerned with what we don't have. Our relentless pursuit of external things to make us fulfilled and validated affects our emotional and physical health. It begins insidiously, and we are unaware of how we are playing into the hands of "events" and "situations," allowing them to decide how we should be.

The aim is to deal with priorities in life but, at the same time, remain consciously aware of our own selves. We are used to many role-playing. Those are our responsibilities, but our primary responsibility lies in knowing ourselves. It helps us to be at peace with what happens around us while we continue fulfilling our obligations.

Yoga means *union*. We feel connected with our inner selves and with our surroundings here and now. We become aware of our breaths, their effects on body parts, and how our body is aligned with the environment. We understand that change is a certainty. We must learn to accept it and incorporate it within ourselves. The exercises help us to regain our individuality. Our faith in ourselves helps us care for our physical and emotional health. Thus, yoga combines physical, mental, and spiritual healthcare practices, resulting in a state of harmonious existence.

The *asana*s cleanse the body by improving blood flow and regulating hormone secretions and functions. Together with *pranayama,* they help to remove stress and side effects of chronic diseases like high blood pressure, type 2 diabetes, asthma, obesity, and overweight.

Stress and anxiety cause chemical imbalances in the body. Yoga sees our bodies and minds as a seamless connection. Thus, it is natural for the stress of daily life to affect our physical as well as mental health, causing anxiety, depression, or sometimes aggression. Yoga works to correct these imbalances to restore complete health.

Vyadhi, or disease, according to yoga master Patanjali is due to mental disturbances, *citta-vrittis*, and it is only through mindfulness techniques that we can become aware of our wrong ways of looking at things, question our beliefs and assumptions, and gain the courage to look at things from a newer, and healthier perspective.

The principal aim of yoga is to guide our minds back to our naturally poised state, where we are alert and curious about our environment without being judgmental. We develop clarity of thought and profound understanding. Our knowledge makes us more compassionate to ourselves and others. We become more accepting and empathic.

Clarity of mind evokes spirituality and trust. Most of our woes stem from a lack of a sense of belonging to the world's happenings. Yoga asanas reestablish why and how we are all parts of the main, not mere islands left on our own. It gives us comfort and peace. We are inspired to live each day to the fullest and root our happiness in small things that uplift our souls.

The impact of yoga on mental health is so significant that medical professionals developed a new term, medical yoga, to treat psychological conditions. It is using yoga asanas to *prevent* and *treat* mental health problems. Yoga has positive effects on improving the strength, flexibility, endurance, and functions of internal organs. With appropriate breathing techniques, yoga evokes a state of mindful awareness of our bodies in relation to the immediate environment.

Many medical conditions, like type 2 diabetes, high blood pressure, and asthma, are related to stress and are aggravated by it. Yoga relieves stress and reduces disease parameters. It also fortifies mental stamina, instilling positive feelings and lowering aggression, depression, and anxiety (Stephens, 2017).

I became interested in yoga as a holistic therapy based on the tenet of spirituality. As I trained and worked closely with my students, I found how mental issues can upset overall health. I introduced mindful chair yoga techniques for seniors unable to stand for long. I aimed to awaken students' minds and then gently connect them with their bodies as they molded into different asanas. This is therapeutic yoga which scientists believe can establish a holistic healthful state (Woodyard, 2011). The asanas themselves reflect nature and all things natural. Mindfully doing them makes us more aware of our postures concerning the world we see around us.

As we learn to focus more on the present, we develop a profound understanding of why we chose our life path and where we are feeling stuck. It is essential to sort this out because this mental block is the cause of our unhappiness. Counseling may help us ponder our thoughts and feelings, but yoga establishes our minds on an inward path. This inner journey of self-discovery enables us to focus more on appropriate life choices, for we all aim to live happily and stop being at war with ourselves.

Yoga helps us to discover that precious roadmap.

The book on mindful chair yoga is on gentle yoga practices focused on mindfulness, meditation, and improving mental stamina. The book has five chapters. Chapter One discusses mental health problems in women aged 50 - 70 years or over. It is a particularly vulnerable time for women when they suddenly find they are losing youth and vitality. The senses lose their acuity, balance teeters, gait falters, and even the mind is not as sharp as it used to be. Any physical or mental trauma during this time is difficult to heal. Still, we endeavor to remain courageous and hopeful. We seek ways to stay focused on good things in our lives. In that vein, the second chapter is on managing mental health conditions, both preventative and curative.

The third chapter is on positive mindfulness, mindful yoga, and its therapeutic effect on our well-being. The beauty of yoga is its ability to enable us to find ways to cure. Yoga gurus insist that yoga is a mere method. *You* are really empowering *yourself* to feel better again, both inside and out.

Chapters four and five are dedicated chair yoga asanas to improve mental health, attention, present moment awareness, and mental stamina. Even 10 minutes of consistent practice can improve mental wellness.

Let us begin our journey together on this path to self-rejuvenation.

Chapter One

Mental Health in Women

"Peace begins with a smile."

- Mother Theresa

The World Health Organization (WHO) describes health as "a state of complete physical, mental, and social well-being and not merely the absence of disease and infirmity."

Mental health means we are emotionally, psychologically, and socially well-adjusted and comfortable. It implies we have analytical and perceptive capabilities in understanding ourselves and others and can regulate our thoughts and feelings. We can question our beliefs to determine their validity under changing circumstances. We know we cannot always behave according to our emotions and must leave room for the bigger picture to fill in the gaps.

Thoughts are more automatic and cannot be prevented. But thoughts can overestimate the adversity or negativity of a particular situation. Instinctive reactions based on thoughts can be regrettable. An individual with sound mental health uses cognition to understand the justification of thoughts and feelings before deciding a course of action.

Cognition is brain power and involves focus, intelligence, memory, judgment, and the capability to assess a situation correctly. It also means understanding and knowing the language and culture of the individuals we interact with daily.

Good mental health gives us a general feeling of well-being and happiness. It reflects on our physical health, behavior, and actions. We enjoy our relationships and social engagements. We show interest in day-to-day happenings, care for our health and sleep well at night.

We often use the term *holism* in lifestyle practices. Lifestyle choices affect our outlook, values, and preferences. In that vein, healthy lifestyle choices like healthy nutrition, healthcare, exercise, and education can all upgrade our health and vitality.

As a lifestyle approach, holism encompasses all aspects of life. It includes alternative medicine and alternative forms of exercise like yoga to enhance our energy and preserve our health.

Holism fosters positive mental health. We create a healthy work-life balance. It makes us feel less nervous and agitated. We are more in control of our lives.

Causes of Stress in Women

The cause of stress in women can be the same as men's, like careers, health, financial constraints, mortgages, and relationship issues.

Other causes are unique to women. They are related to their different roles as wives, mothers, sisters, colleagues, or friends. Traditionally, women are caregivers for their families. Women dedicate more time to family than men. They worry more about elderly parents, siblings, and children. The nature of caregiving activities is entirely different from workplace load and obligations. Managing two and sometimes more roles with perfection can be demanding. Working to fulfill all targets within time can be overwhelming. It becomes even more excruciating when these loads are persistently present. Pressures to meet time constraints and obligations may spur a deep sense of failure.

Meeting others' expectations or our demands of ourselves leaves us little time to self-care. We don't have enough time for self-grooming, let alone care for paying attention to *why* we are stressed.

Women perceive things differently than their male counterparts; they tend to internalize and ruminate about events and situations, seeking emotional explanations. While men look at things more practically, women judge things emotionally. Hence, disorders like depression, anxiety, and eating disorders are more common in women. Some other conditions are unique in women and involve major life transitions like transition into womanhood, pregnancy, childbirth, and menopause.

These periods are associated with hormonal changes. Shifts in the levels of female hormones like estrogen and progesterone can cause mood changes. As women, most of us have undergone premenstrual fog— besides the usual bloated-up feelings— leading up to the days of actual menstruation. It appeared as an inability to concentrate, forgetfulness, and faltering with decision-making processes. Some have more severe premenstrual dysphoric disorder, affecting mood.

Pregnancy is related to anxiety and depression. So is the postpartum period. After childbirth, many of us have grappled with depression and intense fear of inadequacy. However, for most of us, approaching menopause comes as a shock.

Menopause and Mental Health

Menopause is a time when women undergo a major change in their reproductive life cycle. Hormonal levels like estrogen and progesterone decline, and metabolism slows down. Effects of these changes are on the reproductive organs, bones and muscles, thyroid glands, and the heart.

But while these changes are physical, the mental excursions of menopause are more debilitating for many. Headaches, night sweats, and palpitations prevent restful sleep at night. We may wonder at our remarkable transformation. The following psychological experiences can occur during menopause:

- Dizziness

- Anxiety
- Inability to focus
- Irritability and mood swings
- Aggression
- Loss of interest in sexual activities
- Depression

Pre-existing mental health conditions such as schizophrenia and bipolar disorders can worsen during menopause (Szelgia, 2021). Individuals prone to anxiety and stress may experience worsening symptoms during this vulnerable lifecycle.

Approaching the cessation of our reproductive lifecycle is disconcerting and raises stress, fear, and anxiety. And it is not limited to hormonal changes; we also worry more about our children, spouses, or partners and getting older. We tend to gather more information from several sources, many unreliable, thus, increasing our fears.

Chronic stress and anxiety work in a vicious cycle. The more we worry about the unknown, the more it entraps us in its twisted maze. We may have breakdowns over trivia and feel embarrassed at our weaknesses after. Persistent mental anguish can affect life in totality. Things we enjoyed doing no longer seem worthwhile. We interact less socially and spend our days indoors, choosing a sedentary existence over actions like exercises and social engagements. Our choices make us even more isolated and feel lonely.

A dispirited lifestyle affects the health and vitality of the whole body. It also fosters negative self-belief, anger, guilt, and feelings of worthlessness. We sleep inadequately and poorly, lose appetite, or overeat. Mental issues undermine proper judgment, decision-making, and memory.

Positive Psychology

Positive psychology, which is integral to yoga, is centered around the concept of well-being. Our aim is to determine factors that will improve our well-being. As a concept, it is often subjective, with positive and negative implications. For instance, we may choose to eat oily or sugary foods believing they are required for our feelings of well-being. We may choose to ignore physical training because we do not consider it to contribute to our feelings of wellness.

Hence, well-being is an individual choice, and we are obligated to discover activities that are meaningful to us and foster healthy relationships with others. A reciprocatory relationship encourages well-being, otherwise called the "quality of life." Even when we suffer from mental issues, we mostly want to escape them. The trouble is, we do not know how to. The way out for all of us is to improve our emotional intelligence and mental stamina.

Effects of Stress

We experience stress at different life transitions. Stress can be developmental, educational, or social. Factors like career, financial constraints, grief, and trauma can be stressful. Mental health professionals believe that our perception of stress levels and our ability to control it determines our mental resilience.

Psychological resilience refers to emotional and behavioral abilities to remain calm during periods of crisis or chaos. We can manage our emotions and move forward without allowing adverse circumstances to create lasting repercussions.

Stress and crisis momentarily blind us to our choices, decision-making, and actions. Chronic stress can upset our sense of mental balance.

But stress has a good effect as well. We learn to develop emotional resilience by handling myriads of stressful factors we encounter every day. The more successfully we resolve an issue, the better the feedback we give ourselves regarding our ability to manage stress.

Not all of us can manage the same level of stress. While some can find extreme stress levels stimulating, it can throw many others into disarray.

We can only manage stress when we engage with it. Since stress affects our mental, spiritual, and physical states—the classical iron-triad—to avert or manage stress, we must engage with all of them in a coordinated and coherent manner.

Why Yoga is Best?

Yoga is the best method that engages our physical, mental, and spiritual energies to deepen our understanding of ourselves and others. It gives us the rare "how-to" to manage stressful situations more to our advantage.

Yoga is also the best method for enjoying a restful sleep.

Stress disrupts sleep for many. But seniors need the same amount of sleep for 7 - 8 hours as others do.

Lack of sleep makes us irritable and more depressed. Chronic sleep deprivation can cause fatigue, poor concentration, and, often, forgetfulness.

Insomnia or lack of sleep becomes more common after 60 years. You have trouble falling or staying asleep. You may wake up very early without feeling refreshed. It can last for days or even months.

Yoga practices like breathing techniques and meditation are calming and deeply relaxing. Some asanas can help you to sleep better at night.

Positive Mindfulness

Mental health is foundational to collective as well as individual well-being. Emotionally intelligent individuals think, adapt, and interact with others so that everyone can enjoy a good life. On this ground, its promotion, restitution, and conservation become vital to all of us.

Summary

Health is defined by WHO as "a state of complete physical, mental, and social well-being and not merely the absence of disease and infirmity."

Good mental health lets us control our behaviors and actions and make suitable life choices.

Psychological changes can occur during menopause.

Yoga is the best method to utilize and strengthen our physical, mental, and spiritual energies to live a better life.

In the next chapter, we will discuss the management of stress in women in the age group of 50 - 70 and above.

Chapter Two

Stress And Management of Stress in Women of Age Group Fifty to Seventy And Above

"When things change inside you, things change around you."

- Anonymous.

What is Stress?

Stress is our responses, both internal and external, to daily events and experiences— the effects of how we respond to stress fall on our behaviors and actions. Internal stress unsettles the body's finely-tuned organ functions.

We all experience stress in daily life. Some amount of stress keeps us motivated in our work. We can finish deadlines, for example. But continuous stress is harmful and distressing. It frazzles our nerves; we feel demotivated and exhausted.

For many of us, stress builds up due to several factors and reaches a point when we can no longer cope. It almost becomes a part of our existence. We cannot *afford to* slow down yet get overwhelmed by stress. It is like riding on a tiger's back— a perfect catch-22 situation— when you have agreed to do something you cannot let go of.

It takes many breakdowns and general deterioration of health to make us aware of how stress negatively affects our lives. Timely diagnosis and management can, undoubtedly, prevent troubles afterward. But how do we know that we are stressed?

Symptoms of Stress

Stress can produce many symptoms. Women may have different features than men of their corresponding age group. In women, we can find tension affects the following areas.

Physical

Physical symptoms of stress manifest in unique ways. They are nonspecific and difficult to ascribe to health conditions. Hence, you may overlook them.

Unlike specific diseases, we do not experience symptoms like temperature due to infection, typical pains due to organ inflammation and infections, or diarrhea due to stomach infestations.

The symptoms can be any of these features but more subtle in their expressions. Thus, we can have loose motions or constipation as a component of irritable bowel syndrome, which is stress-related.

Stress can cause digestive problems, skin problems, palpitations, headaches, generalized body aches and pains, fatigue, and sleeplessness despite being overly tired. They can happen in many disease conditions as well.

These symptoms can be, therefore, misleading. For instance, tiredness and lack of energy can be due to anemia or thyroid dysregulation, both medical conditions and treatable with medications.

This is why you may be advised to conduct several investigations to arrive at a conclusive diagnosis.

Stress can lead to overeating or losing appetite, smoking, misusing drugs or alcohol, and falling interest in things you enjoy doing.

Emotional

Stress is overwhelming. Somewhere deep within, we know we have too much to deal with effectively, but our conscience tells us to egg on. Sometimes we assume that others would fail to understand our problems and it is better to keep it to ourselves. Explaining our feelings and emotions is difficult, even to close relationships. Bottled-up emotions lead to nervousness, irritability, an irresistible sense of losing control over situations and experiences, and unhappiness. We become more anxious and agitated. We show frustration when things do not happen our way. If we are in perimenopausal or menopausal phases, we may experience debilitating mood swings.

Mental

The mental effects of stress affect cognition and executive functions. Cognition is high-level brain functioning. The area of our brain that controls cognition is the most actively working region. It is called the frontal cortex, and it resides in the front part of the brain. The frontal cortex regulates activities like logical thinking, reasoning, and understanding before responding to what we experience or see daily.

We make our frontal cortex work hard by making innumerable decisions, some necessary, others incidental, or overly regulating our social behaviors. It is energy-consuming, and the brain cells are one of the highest energy users of the body. Consequently, its performance falls. Persistent stressful situations can cause "cognitive overload." Similar conditions happen when we multitask due to time constraints. Or maybe because we cannot say "no" effectively to others.

Since cognition deals with essential functions like memory, problem-solving, picking up social cues, and sensing environmental conditions, chronic stress affects healthy mental functioning. We become inattentive, forgetful, tensed, and sometimes bored.

Profession

Stress affects our careers and professional lives. In workplace situations, we may take longer to finish work, meet deadlines, or miss them. We complain of work overload, fall out with our colleagues or boss, and behave rudely with clients or customers. We make mistakes and feel annoyed with our output. Our careers seem unfulfilling, and we feel stuck.

Social

Stress saps our energy. We avoid people or intimate relationships and complain about being lonely. We avoid social gatherings and commitments, excusing ourselves by citing unsatisfactory or flimsy reasons. In its turn, social isolation amplifies our stress and anxiety.

Spiritual

Spirituality makes us feel peaceful in our lives. It gives us hope and comfort. We draw on our spiritual resources during troubled times. We remain calm as we go through various life experiences. The meaning of spirituality can be different for all of us. Some of us may find support in nature, yet others believe in god and the power of prayer.

Chronic stress affects spiritual health. We lose the only belief system or faith to support our life situations. We may have a mind to let go of our faith. Spirituality keeps us afloat during stress. It is what keeps us whole. Losing it hastens the loss of mental balance only.

Loss of spirituality causes numbness of feelings, loss of meaning in life, self-doubts, an unforgiving attitude, guilt, and hopelessness.

Management of Stress

Stress management begins with self-awareness. We must stop and reflect on why we are feeling overwhelmed. It involves carefully scrutinizing different areas of our lives and understanding how they affect our mental health.

Self-care routines are crucial to self-preservation and maintain a healthy balance in life.

While self-examining the probable causes for stress, consider all six areas of functioning, physical, emotional, mental, professional, social, and spiritual.

Consider how you would like your life to be. At sixty, most of us would agree to live a satisfactorily healthy life. We would like to enjoy strong relationships and good social interactions. We may also want to let go of our past and move forward. We want to enjoy the sunshine every day and greet our neighbors with a smile.

Defining how different you would like your life to be from the present helps you to focus on the stress factors. While it may not be possible to overcome all of them, you can organize your workload and expectations to feel more relaxed.

Stress alleviation involves managing all six life areas.

Physical

Exercise, relaxation techniques, yoga, and meditation all help to reduce stress. Eat healthy foods. Drink plenty of water. Reduce alcohol consumption and stop smoking. Smoking causes sleep deprivation and agitation. Getting enough sleep at night is vital to a healthy lifestyle.

Emotional

Expressing emotions is crucial to making others see and understand your perspectives. Tell others about your feelings clearly and emphasize what you expect from them.

Make a habit of writing a journal. You can use it in different ways. Journaling can help you plan and organize your work for the day, make provisions for relaxation and hobbies, and reveal issues that need urgent attention. You can prioritize your work accordingly.

Love, tenderness, and empathy are positive emotions. Any action that lifts up our hearts is positive. Responding to a neighbor's greetings with a smile is also positive. When you experience a positive emotion, try to be with it and seek ways that will give you similar joys.

Respect yourself and expect no less from others. Relationships based on mutual respect create positive bonds.

Mental

Mental resilience or stamina depends on emotional intelligence. Have a realistic attitude to life, accept how things are at present, and become creative to discover ways to stay better.

Professional

Careers need overhauling and attention from time to time. Organize your workload, identify areas of work-life balance, and set limits on both. Consider a hybrid or a part-time profession to have more time for your family and yourself.

Social

Foster loving relationships, set and maintain healthy boundaries, and stay socially connected. The current emphasis on virtual connection can never substitute physical, social interactions. Simple acts of going out with your friends and families and spending a day in the sunshine are mentally refreshing and energizing.

Spiritual

We seek a meaningful connection with something bigger than ourselves. It evokes *positive emotions, like* awe, delight, gratitude for abundant joy and hope in nature's creation, and acceptance of any shortcomings in our lives. We stop instant negative appraisal of things and look at things more openly and kindly.

Professional Help

Seek professional help for managing significant anxiety, panic attacks, or depression. Medications and behavioral therapy like cognitive behavior therapy can elevate mood, reduce depression, and improve emotional health.

Summary

Some amount of stress keeps us motivated in our work.

Chronic stress can produce many symptoms affecting overall health.

Stress affects six domains of life, physical, emotional, mental, occupational, social, and spiritual.

To manage stress, we must focus on all these six aspects of life.

The next chapter is on mindfulness, how it reduces stress, and yoga's role in improving mindfulness, reducing stress, restoring calmness of the mind, and improving sleep.

Chapter Three

Positive Psychology, Mindfulness, And Yoga

"Mindfulness means paying attention in a particular way, On purpose, in the present moment, and non-judgmentally."

- Sridhar.

Mindfulness is focusing on our present moment to experience what is happening around us without being judgmental. It means that we do not attempt to explain our experiences with our feelings and emotions. We do not use our past experiences of similar situations to estimate their meaning.

Our natural instinct is to compare events, situations, and experiences with past consequences. We use these outcomes to alert us to a possible rerun of the same circumstances. Doing so makes us instinctual and habitual. We depend on general themes, forgetting the subtle changes in the details of every situation.

Our tendency to respond to situations without much thinking has one major fault. We overlook that every case is new, and looking at problems honestly makes us curious and open to learning.

Life is a learning experience, and our past experiences are there to teach us about our responses to situations, not the situations themselves.

Situations will change and sometimes go out of control. We can do nothing about them. The more we try to control problems, the more frustrated, agitated, and stressed we will be.

Instead, we may focus on the events and situations as if they are happening for the first time in our lives. We can go through the experiences carefully and understand them concerning the bigger picture. We can then process them using our past responses. We may remember the effects of our past behaviors and actions on our mental health to better respond in the present moment.

However, for now, we may start only by being mindful of our present moment without judging them.

It is challenging to focus on one thing and guide our minds to shift from moment to moment with precision. It requires patience, discipline, and conscious willpower. At every point of the action, we may catch ourselves thinking laterally, judging situations and people, or trying to color them with our points of view.

Mindfulness

Mindfulness is, therefore, a skill. It is also a *way of being* (Bishop et al., 2004). The good point is, like most skills, we can train ourselves in mindfulness. It will require focus and a change in attitude.

We can improve attention, or focus, by becoming aware of what happens around us daily and how they affect our senses and arouse thoughts and feelings. We also pay attention to the body's responses to external events.

While these are more straightforward ways of practicing mindfulness, we can also practice *meditation* to improve mental concentration.

How can mindfulness help us in self-control and remaining calm in problematic situations?

Scientists have found that a daily mindfulness practice for a prolonged duration improves concentration, self-control on attention, and better awareness of both internal and external experiences.

We can prevent mental excursions, which our elders characterized as "daydreaming." We can hold our focus more on our surroundings and our body's responses to the happenings. For instance, we become more aware of how our heart fills with joy when our children or grandchildren visit us or when our garden flowers bloom. We may find the same peace of mind when reading a book, sewing, or listening to music.

We stop reacting automatically as we teach ourselves a more balanced outlook on external events. We pause to think before we behave, talk, or act.

Mutually beneficial communication is based on respect, trust, and openness. We gradually change our old habits with better-adjusted ones. Our improved responses derive better reactions from others. We understand others' viewpoints and constraints. We know what we can expect from others and ourselves without harming collective interests. We know where we should let go. We can also make others see our perspectives.

Our actions and their effects on others and the situations make us feel good and appreciated. The feeling pervades our physical, emotional, mental, and spiritual domains and positively affects the other two vital areas, social and professional.

A peaceful mind is a mind that is aware of the truth that the capacity to heal ourselves is within us. It restores inner balance and calmness. We are more relaxed, engaged, empathic, and forgiving in a calm mental state. We sleep better at night when our minds are unloaded.

According to the yoga guru Patanjali, the author of the compendium *Yoga Sutras*, a calm mind is on its mark and rests in its rightful position, its actual state of being.

Thus, the sutra 1.3 of the Samadhipada by Patanjali mentioned,

Tada drashtuh swarupe awasthanam,

It means that once we clear our minds of cluttering thoughts, we calm our minds. This is the true state of a yogi when the reasoning mind is consonant with the body and soul. We become curiously aware with an attitude to learn and grow emotionally and mentally.

Research shows that mindfulness reduces stress and creates a feeling of well-being by improving the following aspects of functioning:

- Emotional resilience
- Cognition
- Work engagement and performance
- Social behaviors
- Improved relationships

As a stress-lowering tool, mindfulness training can reduce depression or anxiety and is thus, a protective mental resource (Bartlett et al., 2021).

Mental Resilience

Resilience offers us the mental grit to persevere in the face of setbacks or challenges in life, like losing a job, ill health, or any other disaster. It does not remove our problems. It helps to restore our faith in ourselves and the overall goodness of things, which keeps us motivated during troubled times.

A lack of Resilience makes us weak and vulnerable. We feel overwhelmed, stressed, and unable to cope with situations. We stop looking at the resources we have to regain control of our lives.

Like mindfulness, emotional Resilience helps us to be more optimistic. When we encounter adversity or trauma, we all feel a myriad of emotions like grief, anger, fear, and pain. We may feel stuck or unable to go on with our work at home and office.

An emotionally resilient individual will feel all these emotions but will also try to seek methods to get out of the situation. They will call for help if they cannot cope with the stress. The ability to summon support from others is vital to restoring Resilience.

However, an emotionally resilient person does not dwell on the problem once it is resolved adequately.

Mental Resilience allows us to enjoy our lives and work to the fullest. Our attitude toward life protects us from various mental health conditions.

Emotional Resilience is a skill, and like mindfulness, we can learn them to improve our coping ability.

Learning Emotional Resilience and Mindfulness With Yoga

Yoga can help us to focus more attentively on external events and our internal harmony. It improves mindfulness, calms and relaxes our minds, and fosters mental resilience. Yoga is flexible and adaptable, and it is cost-effective, requiring nothing except a place, a mat, a chair, and your time. You can do it anytime and anywhere, indoors or outdoors.

Meditation is a yoga practice that enhances awareness and engagement with the present moment. It also helps in relaxation. We remain deeply alert to things happening but force our minds not to respond to them. We make our minds still. To do so, we focus on breathing, a strategy that reduces tension.

Deep breathing stimulates the parasympathetic nervous system and subdues the sympathetic nervous system--- our body's autonomic nervous system, which gets triggered in response to stress or lack thereof. While the sympathetic nervous system stimulates our response to a fight-or-flight mode, the parasympathetic is calmative. Chronic stress keeps our bodies locked in a perpetual fight-or-flight mode, flooding us with stress hormones. Meditation and deep breathing activate the body's relaxation mode.

Persistent meditation practice improves spiritual health and restores our faith in ourselves and meaningful others. Our body *repairs* better when relaxed, *immune systems* work *vigorously*, offsetting infections and infestations, and we enjoy *a restful sleep*. We gain mental resilience and self-confidence.

Thus, meditation stops negative assessment of things and helps in cognitive restructuring.

Cognitive Restructuring

Looking at things from a different perspective makes it appear less stressful. Psychologists believe that we view adversity more negatively and sometimes with dread than they actually merit. No situation by itself is positive or negative; how we interpret them gives them a connotation, good or bad. Counselors who practice cognitive behavioral therapy can help to see things from a different outlook than yours and reduce mental stress.

Summary

Mindfulness is a skill, and a *way of being*.

We can train ourselves in mindfulness.

Mental resilience gives us grit to persevere in the face of setbacks or challenges.

Mental resilience and mindfulness reduce stress and stree-related health problems.

Yoga promotes relaxation, mindfulness, and reduces stress.

The next chapter is on asanas that improve attention, breathwork and provide mental relaxation.

Chapter Four

Asanas to Reduce Stress

" Yogaha chitta vritti nirodhah."

- Sutra 1.2.

Samadhipada

The principal aim of yoga is to restore us to a calm mental state. The second sutra of Samadhipada, written by yoga guru Patanjali, states: *"Yogaha chitta vritti nirodhah."*

The sutra implies that we use yoga to reduce mental clutter and distractions.

It is possible because, with yoga, our minds are free from confusion and agitation. We are more grounded and firm in our convictions and abilities. We change our habitual thinking modes and learn helpful adaptations to adjust to our surroundings or circumstances. Thus, the first stage of yoga practice is *arambhavastha, or being at peace.*

Yoga and Nourishment

Yoga considers we are what we eat. Texts in the *Upanishads* clearly state that food comprises 16 parts, of which 10 are waste, 5 are for producing mental energy, and 1 part is required for intelligence. Any food has three different qualities, *sattvic*, *tamasic*, and *rajasic*.

Sattvic foods include vegetables and fruits and are pure. Rajasic and tamasic foods include spices, onion, garlic, meat, alcohol, and contemporary junk foods and are avoided to reduce stress. Drink plenty of water daily to stay hydrated. Water also removes toxins from the body.

The Iyengar yoga believes that stress-relieving yoga can be active or passive. Active postures are traditional poses that are done standing; passive process involves using props like chairs and improves mental calmness and endurance.

Use a stable chair without armrests to do the postures. Wear loose but not overflowing outfits. Keep room temperatures at moderate levels. You can turn on relaxing music as you practice the asanas.

Warm-Up Asanas

All yoga asanas start with warm-ups. They improve muscle mobility and blood flow, making the actual poses easier.

- Sit tall in a chair away from the chair's back.
- Roll your shoulders 10 times, first in one direction and then in another.
- Make neck movements sideways and up and down.
- Make easy kicking movements with your legs.
- Move your arms side-to-side and back and forth a few times.
- Once you feel easy joint movements, you can start with the asanas.

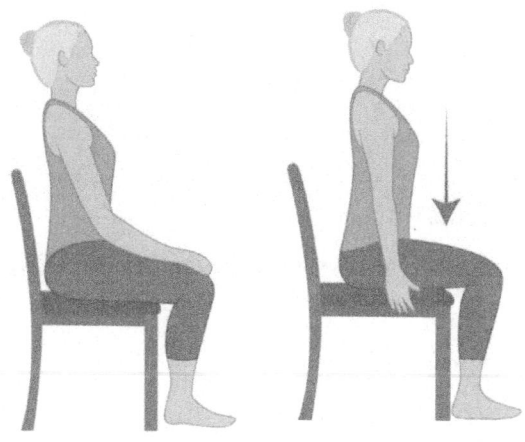

Tadasana Samasthiti

Calming

This asana lifts the heart chakra to reduce stress. The term samasthiti means you remain focused and steady in the upright pose.

Method

- Sit tall in a chair, your back away from the chair's back.
- Your feet must be on the floor, heels touching each other.
- Stretch your arms by your sides as much as possible, your palms must face the thighs and the fingers directed toward the floor.
- Stretch your neck, but keep it soft and relaxed.
- Roll your shoulders back, and lengthen your body.
- Pull in your belly and lift your chest as you inhale deeply.
- Look straight ahead and breathe deeply, in and out.
- Relax the facial muscles.
- Hold your mind still and focus on your breathing.
- Continue for 30 seconds.
- Release.

Forehead Stretch

Relaxing

- Sit upright on the chair.
- Place the index fingers of both hands below the hairline in the center of the face.
- Place your thumbs above the eyebrows.
- Move the fingers away from the center, massaging your skin *gently* but *firmly*.
- While massaging, try to lift your eyebrows, maintaining the tautness of the skin.

- Repeat the massage 4 - 5 times.
- Hold the last stroke in position for 5 seconds.

Eye Stretches

Relaxing

Regular eye stretches can prevent eye bags and lift your cheeks. The movements are deeply relaxing.

Method

- Sit upright on a chair.
- Your index fingers should be on the outer corners of your eyes.
- Your second fingers are on the inside corners of the eyes.
- Gaze up toward the eyebrows, keeping the forehead relaxed.
- Release.
- Repeat 5 - 10 times.

Cheek Massage

Relaxing

- Now place your thumbs underneath the cheekbones, flanking your face with them.
- Curl your lower lip around the teeth of the lower jaw.
- Exert a little pressure with your thumbs, smile, and lift your cheekbones.
- Repeat the pose four times.
- On the fifth time, hold the pose for 5 - 10 seconds.

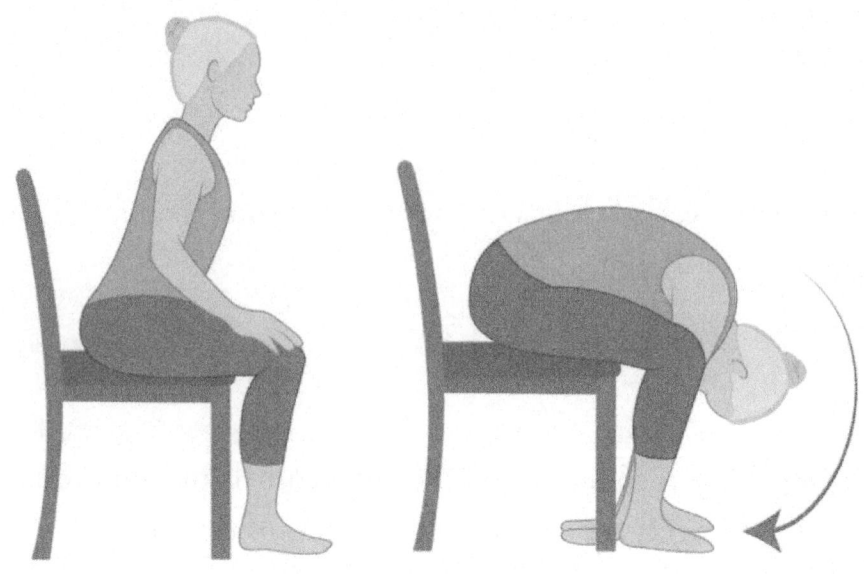

Folding Forward Bending Pose

Calming & Stretching

The prasarita padattonasana in Sanskrit is the foundational or base pose of the Iyengar yoga school. It is a beginner-level yoga pose.

Method

- Sit on a chair, your back away from the chair's back. Your feet rest on the ground, at hip-width apart.
- Spread your feet widely, as far as you can. The toes must point slightly outward.
- Inhale deeply, opening your chest.
- Exhale and fold forward from your waist, bending your head down.

- Bring your hands on the floor just below the shoulders. Alternatively, you may rest them on or around the shins.
- Your head must be between your thighs.
- Soften the knees and your neck.
- Feel the deep stretch in the back and the leg muscles.
- Breathe gently in and out of the posture for 5 - 8 breaths and release.

Benefit

- Stretch the hamstrings, calves, lower back, hips, and back.
- Relaxing for the body.

Contraindication

- Avoid the posture in the following conditions:
- Hernia
- Groin, knee, or back pain
- Spinal disc injury
- Unregulated blood pressure
- Dizziness
- Glaucoma
- Retinal detachment

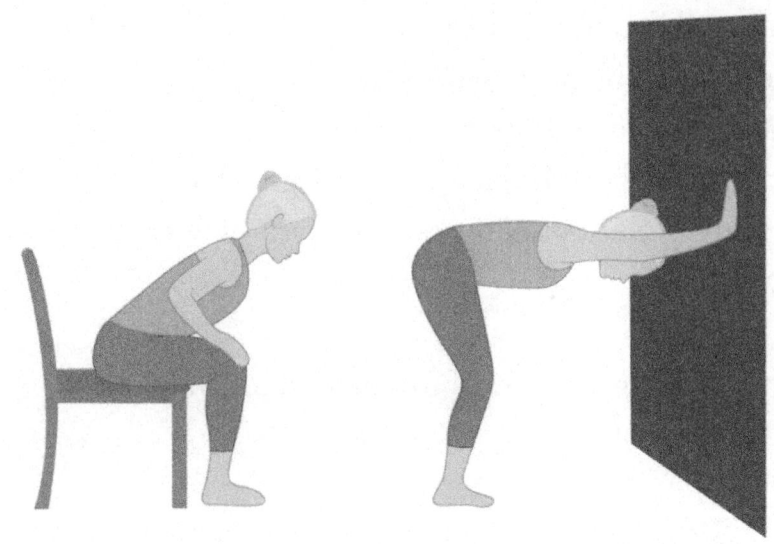

Half-Forward Wall Bend Pose

Calming

Also called Ardha Uttanasana, this pose is done standing, but we will use a chair for our purpose.

Method

- Place the chair about one foot away from a wall.
- Sit on the chair, your back away from the chair's back. Keep your feet hip-width apart.
- Inhale deeply.
- Exhale and bend at your waist to rest your hands on the wall. Your palms must be at hip level.
- Your back must be straight and parallel to the floor.
- Press down on the floor and breathe deeply in and out of this pose for 30 -60 seconds.

- You can adjust the distance of the chair from the wall to feel a better stretch in your back,
- Keep your neck relaxed throughout the pose.

Benefit

- It lengthens the back.
- Stimulated organ functions.
- Relaxation to the whole body.

Contraindication

- Injury to the shoulder muscles.

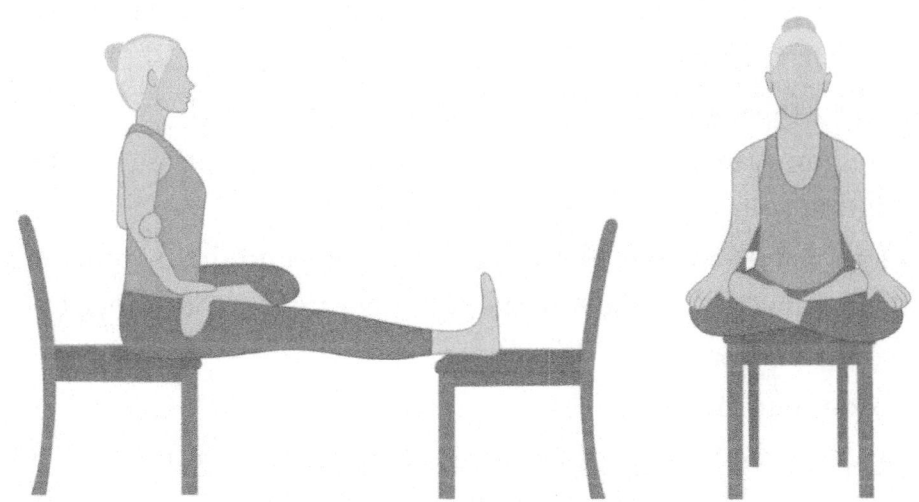

Lotus Pose

Calming

Lotus pose, or Padmasana, opens up your body like a budding lotus. It is a meditative pose. It is an intermediate-level pose.

Method

- Choose a chair with a wide seat to accommodate a folded-legged position. A chair without an armrest would be the best choice. Alternatively, use a low bench or a couch.
- Sit with your legs stretched forward if you sit on a couch; keep your legs on the mat if you choose a chair to do the asana.
- Raise the right knee, placing it on the left thigh. The sole must point upward, and the heel must be closer to your body.
- Raise the left leg and place it on the right thigh similarly.
- You are now seated, with your legs crossed, your feet on the thighs, and the soles facing you.
- Rest your hands on your thighs; you can make a mudra by touching the tips of the forefingers with the thumbs and other fingers spread open.
- Lift your chin and chest.
- Roll back your shoulders.
- Inhale deeply and exhale slowly for 5 - 8 breaths and relax.
- Beginners can do a half-lotus pose by positioning one leg on the thigh at a time.

Benefits

- Reduces muscular tension and lowers blood pressure.
- Relaxes the mind
- Aids digestion

Contraindication

- Ankle or knee injury or surgery.

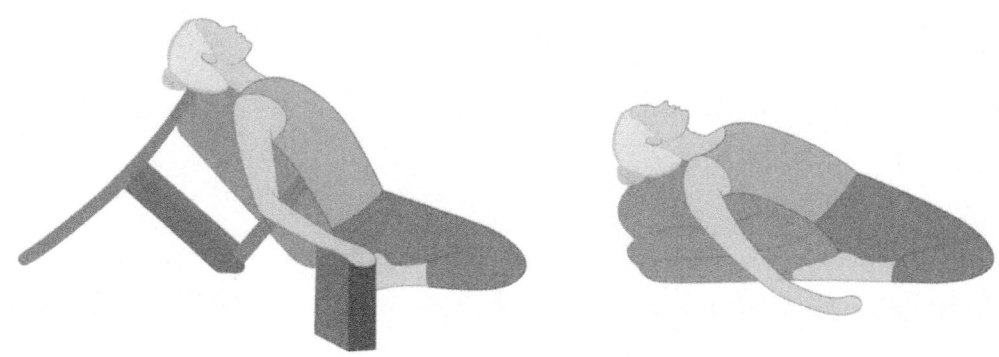

Reclining Hero

Relaxation

Reclining hero or supta virasana is done reclining. It is advanced-level yoga, especially if you are using a couch to do the pose. You can use a chair or a couch to do the asana.

You will need a bolster for the yoga. You can also stack pillows for reclining.

Place the bolster or the stack of pillows on the backside of the chair. Although this is a reclining pose, you must not overstretch your body backward.

Method

- Sit on the front side of a chair. Ensure that you are sitting on your tailbone.
- Keep your feet firmly on the ground if you are using a chair.
- If you use a couch, kneel on your shin bones, and separate your ankles to sit between them. Keep your knees wide. Your legs must be folded behind your back.

- Now, recline back on the bolster, resting your back. Support your head on a pillow or a blanket.
- Breathe deeply in the pose, holding it for 30 - 60 seconds.

Benefit

- Deeply relaxing
- Strengthening of body.
- Promotes digestion.

Contraindication

- Doing the pose by folding your legs behind your back can be challenging. Use the chair for a more easy pose.

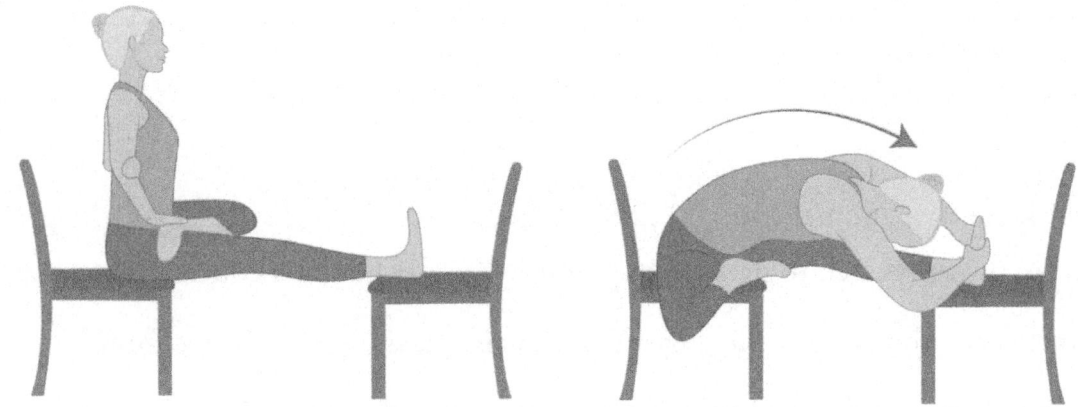

Head-to-Knee Pose

Relaxing

Janu Sirasana, or head-to-knee pose, is a relaxing and stretching yoga pose. Use chairs or a couch for the asana. Avoid rounding the back in this asana. It is challenging, but you can do it slowly and carefully.

Method

- Sit tall on a stable chair and spread your feet on another chair. You can use a couch. Alternately, you can extend both limbs forward, keeping your heels firmly on the ground. Your legs must be hip-width apart. Feel the stretch at the back of your legs.
- Now bend the right knee outward and rest the sole on your left thigh. If your legs are extended on the ground, you can rest the heel against the left ankle.
- Inhale deeply.
- Slowly fold over on the bent knee as you exhale, keeping your neck and spine long. It is not necessary to dip your head to the knee. Do not round your back.
- Stretch your hands on either side of the leg to support your body, or hold the right sole.
- Feel the stretch in your body as you breathe deep and slow into the pose.
- Hold the pose for 30 - 60 seconds and relax.
- Repeat the pose on the other side.

Benefit

- Stretch the entire body.
- Relaxing.

Contraindication

- Back, knee, or foot injury.

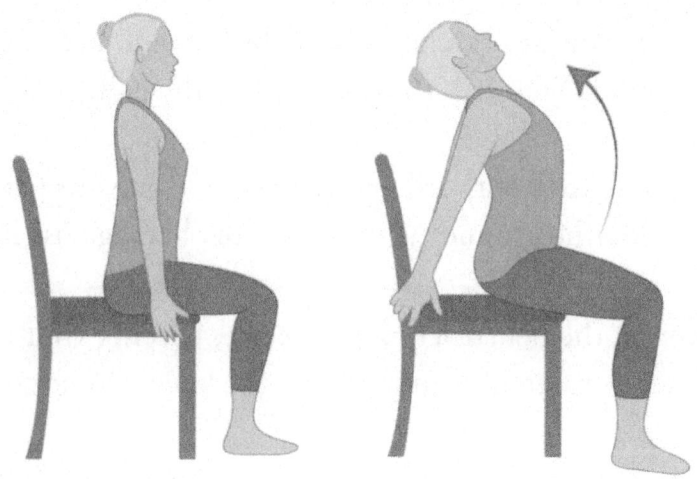

Sphinx Pose Chair Version

Stretching and Relaxing

The pose is called Bhujangasana in Sanskrit. Bhujanga means snake. Hence, the pose is also known as Bhujangasana. It is a beginner asana.

Method

- Sit tall on a chair, your back away from the chair's back.
- Rest your feet firmly on the ground.
- Take your hands back and hold the sides of the chair firmly.
- Inhale deeply, lifting your chin and opening your chest. Look toward the ceiling, keeping an arched back.
- Exhale slowly

- Stay in the pose to feel the stretch in your back and front of the neck for a few more breaths. With each exhalation, feel the deep relaxation of the pose. Allow yourself a smile.

Benefit

- It is energizing for the body and mind.
- Whole body stretching.

Contraindication

- Avoid the asana in injury or surgery of the back, shoulders, and hands.

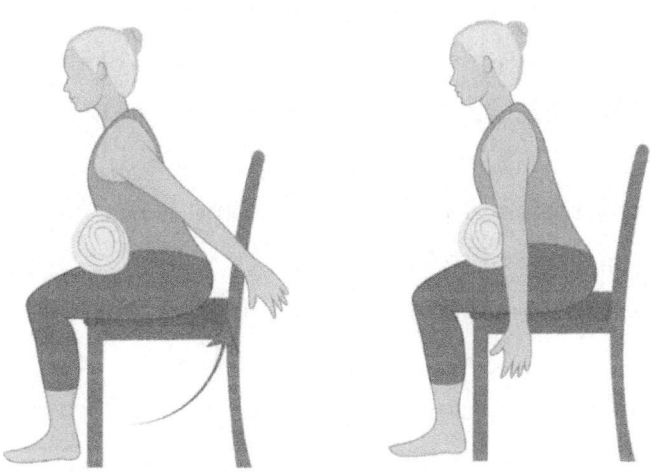

Locust Pose

Relaxing

The locust pose, or salabhasana is a relaxing and stretching asana. This is a beginner pose and is called a baby backbend. It resembles an infant who has just learned to turn on his back.

You will require a folded blanket or a bolster to support your belly for this asana.

Method

- Sit on a chair in a tadasana position.
- Place the folded blanket on your lap.
- Fold forward, placing your belly on the blanket.
- Extend your arms behind your back on both sides of the chair.
- Inhale and lift your chest. Simultaneously, press your belly on the blanket. Your neck must be long, and you gaze at the ground.
- Exhale and lower the chest on the blanket and lower your arms.
- Repeat the asana a few more times.
- On the final round, breathe in and out slowly as you hold the pose for 10 - 20 seconds.
- Return to resting position and breathe for another 10 breaths.

Benefit

- Stretching for the spine.
- Opens your chest.
- Relaxes the body and the mind.
- Promotes sleep.

Contraindication

- Avoid if you have a spine or neck injury.

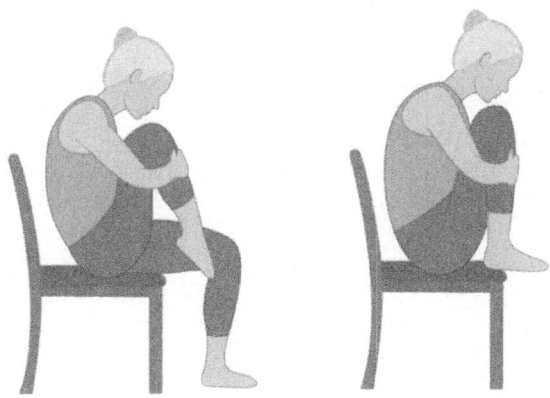

Knees-to-Chest Pose

The Knees-to-chest Pose or apanasana is a beginner asana that relaxes your body and mind. It is a rocking boat motion when done lying on a mat. For our purpose, we will use a chair to sit on it as we do the pose.

Method

- Sit tall on a chair, your back away from the chair's back.
- Stretch your arms by your side.
- Exhale and bring your knees to your chest, clasping them with your arms.
- Loosen your shoulders, and lengthen your spine.
- You can rock to-and-fro in this pose if the chair supports you well.
- Hold the pose for a minute, and breathe easily.
- Release the pose as you exhale.

Benefit

- Improve blood flow.
- Relaxing asana.

Contraindication

- Avoid if you have acute back problems.

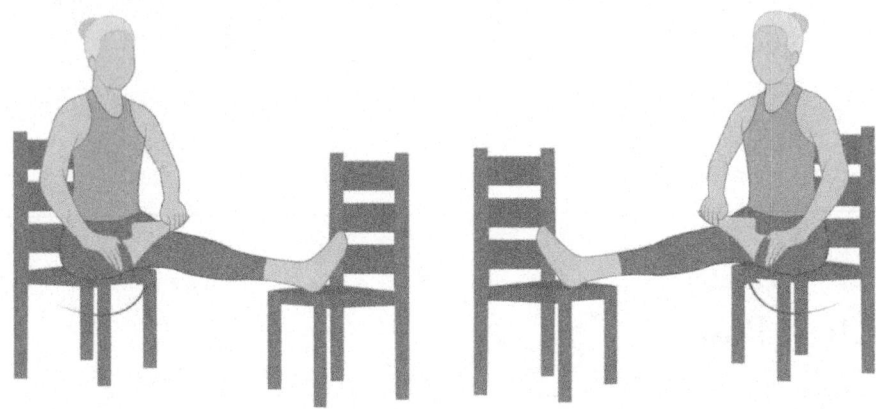

Half-butterfly Pose

Half-butterfly Pose or ardha titliasana is a modification of the full butterfly asana, which is done seated on the mat.

Method

- Sit tall on a chair, your back away from the chair's back.
- Lift your right leg on the left thigh, and support your right knee with your left hand.

- Now flutter the right knee like a butterfly as you breathe in and out of the pose.
- Repeat the asana on the other side.

Star Pose

This is a vinyasa pose in yoga and combines many postures into one.

A stretching and deeply relaxing pose, the star pose is easy to do but intensely relaxing.

Method

- Sit tall on a chair, your back away from the chair's back.
- Spread your feet wide apart, your heels pointing slightly outward.
- Stretch your hands to your side as far as you can.
- Keep your body tall.
- Breathe slowly in and out for as long as you can.
- Release and relax.

Summary

Use a sturdy chair without an armrest to do the yoga.

Begin yoga with a warm-up, and end with a cool-down.

Start practicing the asanas slowly without exerting yourself.

Start with three to four asanas, and repeat them two to three times. Increase the frequencies and repetitions gradually.

The next chapter is on breathing techniques and mindful yoga to help you relax better and sleep well at night.

Chapter Five

Breathing And Mindful Yoga

"When the mind is still, it gets the power to fulfill any thought."
- Ravishankar, Art of Living

Foundation

According to yoga, we have to face and deal with many challenges in our daily life. Most of these minor or significant issues make us tense and uncomfortable. We may not constantly be aware of how our breathing becomes fast and shallow, heart rates increase, fingers curl up into fists, or the forehead wrinkles into a frown. Our body becomes tense, reflecting the inner tension and discomfort.

In yoga, inner tension creates an energy block. Yoga gurus believe energy should flow freely throughout our body, filling every body cell with vitality, called *prana*. An obstacle in the flow of energy flow creates an imbalance of energy. It becomes excess in some parts, dwindling to zero in others. Over time, our body senses energy deprivation and becomes lethargic.

Yoga poses can correct this imbalance of energy. The unique breathing techniques associated with different body movements allow your breath to reach every body part.

You learn to breathe freely and fully, taking in life-giving oxygen while you breathe in. You allow oxygen to reach all your body cells. And, when you exhale, you breathe out fully, expelling air emptied of oxygen. What you breathe out is rich in carbon-di-oxide and is breathed in by the green plants to make food. You contribute beautifully to nature's cycle of life.

When you connect breathing with yoga, you maximize your benefits, cool down your body, and soothe your tensed nerves. Paying more attention to your breaths is not something you do naturally. But when you do, you automatically attempt to slow it down to a more comfortable pace. That is the first step of lowering inner tension.

The benefits of breathwork or pranayama are as follows:

- Developing external and internal awareness.
- Lowering tension.
- Promoting better sleep.
- Enhancing self-cleansing processes of the body.
- Revitalizing our body and mind by restoring the balance between the body and mind.

Pranayama

Prana means life force or vitality. It passes throughout our body through channels called Nadi. There are fixed energy chakras, which are energy centers.

You energize the life force by controlling the length, frequency, and duration of breathing. It consists of three stages, inhalation (puraka), retention (kumbhaka), and exhalation (chakra).

Our mind is calm when the flow of prana is free and smooth. It is important to breathe as you practice pranayama effortlessly.

What You Need

- Do the asanas in a quiet, well-lit corner of your room or outdoors in a peaceful setting.
- Sit on a firm chair or a bench to do the asanas.
- Smile when you do the asanas to help you relax.
- Avoid doing the asanas on a full stomach.

- Doing them in the morning or early evening hours is helpful for energizing the body.
- The breathing sequence is inhalation, hold your breath for 5 seconds and slowly exhale.
- Nadi sodhana pranayama may begin with exhalation.

Bhramari Pranayama

The honey-bee or bhramari pranayama is for beginners.

Method

- Sit straight; when you are ready, close your eyes closed.
- Sit here for a while, noticing the body sensations and the stillness inside you.
- Place your index fingers on the cartilages of the ears.
- Breathe in slowly and deeply.
- Breathe out, *gently* pressing the cartilage. Simultaneously, make a bee-like loud humming sound. You can also apply pressure and loosen it alternately on the cartilage as you make sounds at the back of your throat.
- Keep the pitch high for better results.
- Breathe in and continue to repeat the asana 3-4 times.

Benefit

- Instantly Calming to the body and mind.
- Lowers high blood pressure.

Contraindication

- None.

Kapalbhati Pranayama

In Sanskrit, it means shining skull. It energizes the crown chakra. It is an intermediate to advanced level asana.

Method

- Sit comfortably with your back straight. Your hands are on the knees with palms facing the sky.
- Inhale deeply.
- Pull your belly button back toward the spine as you exhale. Keep your right hand on the stomach to feel the tightening of the belly muscles.
- Relaxing the stomach and the belly button allows air to flow into your lungs automatically.
- Repeat the breathwork 20 times to make a cycle of kapalbhati.
- Relax, close your eyes, and notice the sensations in your body.
- Make two more cycles of kapalbhati.

Benefit

- Of all pranayamas, kapalbhati is the best way to cleanse your body.
- It opens the nadis or the energy channels of the body.

Contraindication

- Having an artificial pacemaker or stent in your heart.
- Hernia.
- Disc prolapse.
- Backache
- High blood pressure.
- Glaucoma.
- Retinal detachment

Bhastrika Pranayama

The bellows breath, or bhastrika pranayama, involves forceful inhalations and exhalations. It is an intermediate to advanced-level asana.

Method

- Sit on a bench or couch with your legs folded under you (Vajrasana). You can sit straight on a chair if you cannot sit in Vajrasana.
- Make a fist and fold your arms and bring them near your shoulders.
- Inhale deeply, simultaneously raise your hands and open your fists.
- Exhale a little forcefully, bring your arms down to your shoulders, and close your fists.
- Repeat the movements sequenced with breathing for 20 breaths.
- Relax, and keep the palms on your thighs.
- Breathe normally.
- Make two more cycles of the asana.

Benefit

- Feel your energy levels rise after three cycles of this asana.
- Stimulates secretion of digestive juices and aids digestion.

Contraindication

- High blood pressure.
- Dizziness.

Nadi Sodhana Pranayama

It is also called alternate nostril breathing, and its purpose is to clean the body channels or nadis. It is a beginner-level asana.

Method

- Sit comfortably on a chair, keep your back straight, and relax your shoulders.
- Close your eyes to feel the effects of the asana.
- Place your left hand on the left knee, opening up the palm. You can also use the chin mudra by touching the index finger with your thumb.
- Place the tip of your right hand's index and middle fingers between your eyebrows, your ring, and little fingers on the left nostril and the thumb on the right nostril. Use the ring and little fingers to open or close the left nostril and the thumb for the right. Use *gentle* pressure
- Press the right nostril with your thumb and breathe out *gently and slowly* through the left nostril.
- Breathe in through the left nostril, and press it gently with the ring and little fingers. Remove your thumb from the right nostril, and breathe out.
- Breathe in from the right nostril and exhale from the left side to make a cycle of nadi sodhana.
- Continue inhaling and exhaling through alternate nostrils.
- Make 9 repetitions.
- After each exhalation, you must breathe in through the same nostril. Hold it and then exhale slowly from the other side. The duration for breathing out should be longer than that of breathing in.

Benefit

- Calming and centering when followed by a 10-minute meditation.
- Powerful deep breathing exercise.
- It balances all three doshas, vata, pitta, and kapha.

Contraindication

- None.

The Pranayama Sequence

You may do the pranayama in the following sequence (What is pranayama and its types & techniques, n.d.).

Bhastrika pranayama

Bhramari prananayama

Nadi shodhana pranayama

Mindful Yoga

Mindful yoga is a relatively new approach to yoga asanas and is based on the principles of Buddhist mindfulness teachings. It opens up awareness and gives an insight into the mind, enabling you to establish a robust and positive mind-body connection. The concept, therefore, is a tool for an improved quality of life.

Do *all your asanas* mindfully to learn how to create inner peace and acceptance.

Method

Before doing any asana, sit tall on a chair, keep your back straight, and close your eyes.

Take a minute here to scan your body.

Open your mind and look for subtle and more obvious ways how your body responds to the thoughts you are having now and how they feel in your body.

Now, start the asana, preserving your sense of selfhood as you change the movements, with an awareness of the feelings each movement brings from moment to moment.

Be curious about what you experience without being judgmental or developing an attachment to what you feel or think.

Then release your focus of attention intentionally and consciously. Shift to another focus of attention as you unfold your body into a new movement. You can make your motions rhythmic like a dance.

Hold each posture for a few seconds to investigate your body and mind's awareness concerning the movement. Breathe evenly.

Being alert and curious like a child is the key to mindful yoga, but never self-critical.

If at any point you find your mind wandering away, notice that, too, without annoyance or judgment. Bring your mind gently back to your breath and the body.

Ask yourself the following questions to derive the full benefit of mindful yoga:

How is your breath, whether shallow or deep? Notice its pace, whether fast or slow.

What is your body's sensation to the poses you are making? Are they mildly painful? Can you bear them? How do the stretches feel? Are they relaxing? Can you stretch your limbs a little more? Would doing that evoke fear? Why?

Where is the sensation arising in the body? How does the sensation feel? Fear, for instance, can feel like a knot in the stomach.

Use the answers to release any negative sensations that you may be feeling. Breathe in and out as you release these knots of sensations and feel deeply relaxed.

Are you in the present or thinking about when this pose will end?

Are you in the present, or are you wondering about something or someone else?

Mindful yoga, like meditation, makes you beautifully aware of your thoughts, feelings, and the sensations these thoughts and emotions produce in your body. Use your input to question what you believe to be true. Mindful yoga helps you notice how thoughts agitate your mind and allows you to unwind.

Conclusion

Therapeutic yoga believes in the application of yoga asanas to manage health conditions. Health is an all-encompassing concept and means the physical, mental, and emotional well-being of an individual. Emotional distress and mental afflictions like anxiety and depression can be as and sometimes even more debilitating than physical conditions. Yoga asanas and postures, together with conscious breathing techniques, reduce anxiety, elevate mood, and synchronize the body, mind, and spirit to make us whole.

We gain strength, vitality, and freshness. Our minds become more aware and open to events occurring in our external and internal worlds. We learn to explore our experiences with our senses and understand our feelings concerning them. The simple techniques reduce our anxiety and make us calmer.

Use the easy approaches of this book to reduce stress and improve your sleep patterns and overall quality of life. The poses have been modified for chair yoga and require 10 minutes of your time. This short time is sufficient to build mental stamina and mindfulness.

Strong Bones for Seniors

Manage and Prevent Osteoporosis. Gentle Targeted Chair Yoga Exercises to Safely Improve Bone Density & Balance

Introduction

"LOVE YOUR BONES: protect your future."

-Theme of World Osteoporosis Day, 2022

At forty-four, Amy did not look like having a condition as grim as osteoporosis. Indeed, those who met her for the first time were surprised to learn that she had it at all. "You don't look like you can have osteoporosis," they said, "You are young and healthy. Isn't osteoporosis a disease of frail older women?"

The stereotypical idea of osteoporosis occurring in underweight postmenopausal women with a family history of osteoporosis precludes women like Amy. She was just thirty when diagnosed, and though not muscled or stout, she was otherwise healthy.

According to Amy, she broke her wrist while she was busy multitasking. It happened so suddenly and unexpectedly that Amy failed to think of a good reason for how it happened. She never had a fall or sustained trauma significant enough to cause a fracture.

Looking back, Amy mused how she always nursed the fear of acquiring osteoporosis sometime in her life. Her mother had the condition, and Amy knew it ran in families. She was mindful of her diet but developed bowel problems when she was 24.

Amy came down with irritable bowel syndrome. She developed a severe allergic response to milk and dairy products. She switched her diet to rice-based products, leaving her diet deficient in vitamin D and calcium. "There is a general lack of awareness," Amy contends, reflecting how important it is to spread the awareness of osteoporosis among women of childbearing age.

Most of us are unaware that our bones are continually renewed and remodeled. Old bone is broken down and is replaced by new bone. The balance is tipped toward bone regeneration up to age 30 when we reach our peak bone mass. After that, the remodeling process slows down, and we lose a little more than we gain. The potential to lose bone mass is 1% each year after age 25 - 30.

But statistics tell us that 80% of older Americans with fractures are not tested or treated for osteoporosis which causes almost 2 million broken bones annually. Approximately 10 million Americans have the condition, and 44 million suffer from low bone density, making them prone to unwarranted fractures.

Gleaning the numbers, we can easily surmise that almost half of all adults at 50 are at increased risk for fractures and should attend to their bone health (Osteoporosis Fast Facts, 2015).

However, the correct age for caring for your bone health starts much earlier, in your twenties or even before.

Osteoporosis can be a serious threat to living independently. Individuals with the condition can break bones after minor trauma or fall. Even straining, coughing, or sneezing can cause bone fractures in more severe conditions.

Women after menopause are more likely to experience osteoporosis owing to the loss of protective hormone actions. Sedentary habits, smoking, alcohol, lack of sunshine, and a diet poor in vitamin D and calcium are other factors that make the bones brittle.

The condition runs in families and usually affects underweight individuals. But, Amy did not squarely fit into any of these stereotypes. She recalled why she should have been more careful about diet supplementation, given that the condition ran in her family. That she did not smoke or drink and walked to her job did nothing to prevent the untimely appearance of osteoporosis when she was barely in her thirties.

"It came as a shock," she mentioned about how she could not believe the doctor's diagnosis after she fractured her wrist. She was in denial for a long time. But the bone scan reports were facts that stared bluntly at her face. At one point, she had to take responsibility for what happened.

Not knowing can be dangerous, but denying an existing condition is irresponsibility and recklessness. Amy stresses discussing osteoporosis with friends and family to spread awareness.

Once you have it, you automatically search for means to minimize the condition's progression. And once you are aware of the possibility of having a condition like osteoporosis later in life, you can take preventative measures to avoid it.

Medical research has progressed considerably in the last decades, and medications previously unknown for checking osteoporosis are now available. Tailored fitness programs help to maintain the bones strong and healthy. Supervised diet modifications and supplementation can improve bone health. Overall, the picture is much better than it was before.

According to Amy, once you know you have dealt with the cards, you accept what happened to you. Acceptance teaches a positive attitude toward life. You know that having a condition is not the end of the road. On the other hand, it is a challenge daring you to live your best no matter the odds.

Many believe the condition cannot be prevented, and no relationship exists between food habits and osteoporosis. But the disease is preventable when you are aware of it and take enough precautions to avoid having it.

Therapy aims at maintaining mobility and strengthening muscles and bones with guided exercise. Diet, vitamin D, and weight-bearing exercises can stop osteoporosis from developing. Once it appears, the same therapeutic protocol, in addition to medications, can halt further bone loss.

For seniors, yoga offers the best choice for low-impact training. You are looking for programs that are safe and supportive. While you can do yoga regularly to improve your strength and balance, you may feel uncomfortable standing for a long time. Chair yoga allows you to do the exercises safely and securely. Simultaneously you benefit from enhancing bone density and maintaining good posture and balance.

Body strength and balance prevent falls and fractures. Chair yoga exercises bolster your ability to deal with osteoporosis with faith and confidence.

The slogan for osteoporosis is "No More Broken Bones." World Osteoporosis Day is celebrated on the 20th of October each year. A theme is adopted for the event to spread awareness of osteoporosis. Individuals and professionals across the medical and related fields discuss and share information on bone health, body postures, the importance of exercise, and diet. People are encouraged to receive diagnosis, treatment, and information on the prevention of osteoporosis.

I have had a long-term connection with yoga; I am passionate about the versatile forms of asanas that efficiently connect the body, mind, and spirit to restore and maintain health and vitality.

While training my senior students, I discovered their anxiety and pain related to body strength, endurance, and balance. I marveled at their spirit to overcome all odds and persist with their functionality. My book will empower all of you looking for ways to improve your bone health by practicing **10-minute** chair yoga postures daily.

The chair asanas are simple but powerful. They are enabling. Live fully by doing these simple asanas regularly, with a healthy diet and lifestyle.

The first chapter is on osteoporosis. You understand the process of bone formation, bone health, and what osteoporosis means for us. You learn why diet, lifestyle, and exercise are vital to bone health.

The second chapter is on the diagnosis of osteoporosis.

The third chapter is on the prevention and management of osteoporosis.

The fourth and fifth chapters discuss several chair yoga postures to prevent and check osteoporosis. The fifth chapter exclusively focuses on strengthening yoga exercises for osteoporosis.

Let us begin our journey into the book by renewing the pledge, "No More Broken Bones."

Chapter One
What Is Osteoporosis?

"People are surprised that I have osteoporosis. Everyone thinks it is a little old lady's disease."

-Susan, osteoporosis patient.

Osteoporosis is Latin for porous bones. It is a bone condition with reduced bone density and bone mass. Sometimes it can happen due to changes in bone structure and strength. Reduced bone vitality makes the bones brittle and vulnerable to sudden fractures.

The surprise element earns osteoporosis its moniker: *Silent disease.* You do not notice that your bones have been weak for a while. You were not even straining when the event took place. Simple postural changes like standing or walking were enough to cause the fracture.

Normal Bone Structure

When we think about bones, we imagine gnarly, pasty-white anatomical structures. They look lifeless. But, despite their looks, bones are active connective tissues of our body that get constantly remodeled and replaced. The process is so consistent that if you considered the whole picture, you would learn that the complete human skeleton gets replaced every 7 - 10 years.

We all know that bones are the structural framework for the muscles, tendons, and ligaments. They enable us to move, bend, and do various other work. Bones also cushion the internal organs from hurt. But bones have other vital functions too.

Bones are storehouses of crucial elements like calcium and phosphorus. The marrow produces blood cells. The bones regulate muscle contractions, nerve signaling, and internal body balance.

All 206 bones of our body have different shapes, sizes, and functions. But they all share a typical internal structure. They have a layer of dense, *compact* bone on the surface. It surrounds a *honeycombed* interior formed by numerous crosshatching lines called trabeculae. It reduces stress, besides providing space for the bone marrow.

Bone Formation

Bones are constructed from a cartilage matrix by the *osteoblasts*, which are bone-producing cells. They lay down collagen on the matrix, absorbing calcium and phosphates from the blood vessels. Calcium phosphate crystallizes on the collagen-cartilage matrix forming the bone structure. The formed bone is 2/3rd protein and 1/3rd mineral.

From fetal life to 25 years of age, the process of bone formation by the osteoblasts surpasses bone-breaking activities by another type of bone cells called the *osteoclasts*. Their actions are not antagonistic but complementary, helping the bone regenerate.

Bone regeneration is necessary to replace structural damage due to constant wear and tear from using skeletal structures for every work we do.

For instance, you ran to catch the train. You succeeded, but the *osteocytes* in your thigh bones detected microscopic tears. The osteocytes are osteoblasts trapped in the bone. They are inactive, but they communicate messages to the osteoblasts and osteoclasts about the requisites for remodeling. It is a highly coordinated process without allowing net changes in bone mass or quality.

In osteoporosis, the honeycomb bone structure is amplified because the bones lose density. Bone mass is reduced. Diminished bone mass and density make the bones unduly fragile.

What Causes Osteoporosis?

When loss of bone mass and density is sufficient to alter bone structure, your bones become soft and brittle. Several causes can affect bone mass, but they don't affect all individuals similarly. Some may get osteoporosis without apparent risk factors. Again, not all risk factors can be avoided. Thus, discussing them will make you aware of the common reasons behind osteoporosis.

- **Age:** Bone loss is more with aging than bone formation, which is slower.
- **Body types:** Thin-built individuals with delicate bone structures are more vulnerable to bone mass loss and fractures.
- **Gender:** Women have a lower peak bone mass and smaller bones than men. With men, the chances of osteoporosis increase after 70.
- **Race:** Non-Hispanic white Americans and Asians are more susceptible to osteoporosis than Hispanic and Afro-American populations.
- **Family history:** The risk of osteoporosis increases if one of your parents has osteoporosis or a hip fracture.
- **Medical conditions:** Associated with adverse bone health include gastrointestinal diseases leading to poor absorption of nutrients, rheumatoid arthritis, some cancers, Acquired Immunodeficiency Syndrome (AIDS), and anorexia nervosa.
- **Diet:** A diet low in calcium and vitamin D can raise the possibility of fractures and osteoporosis. Prolonged dieting or a crash diet lacking essential nutrients and proteins affects bone health poorly.
- **Drugs:** Prolonged use of drugs like proton-pump inhibitors (PPIs), antiepileptic medications, steroids, selective serotonin reuptake inhibitors

(SSRIs), some diabetic medications, and cancer medications can cause bone loss.
- **Lifestyle:** How we live our daily lives, routines, exercises, hobbies, and stress can affect internal health over time. As we age, our unhealthy habits and practices affect organ structures and functions. Besides undermining bone health, lifestyle diseases include metabolic and cardiovascular conditions.

Poor lifestyle choices include the following:

- Sedentary habits and lack of exercise.
- Prolonged heavy drinking.
- Excessive smoking.
- Poor sleep habits.
- **Hormonal factors:** Hormonal levels can alter bone density.
- In women, lowered estrogen after menopause, surgical removal of ovaries, or absent periods due to eating disorders or excessive exercise can affect bone health negatively.
- Prematurely low testosterone can affect bone health more severely than gradually reducing testosterone levels with aging.
- Hyperactivity of the thyroid and parathyroid glands can reduce bone mass.

Who Gets Osteoporosis?

Osteoporosis is found among men and women of all races and ethnicity, although more commonly in women and non-Hispanic whites and Asian populations.

In men, osteoporosis is more common among non-Hispanic whites. African-American and Hispanic Americans, although at risk, have a lesser propensity for osteoporosis.

Unlike the popular concept, it can occur at any age, but its risk increases proportionately. In women, osteoporosis can start developing one to two years before menopause.

Some medications like cancer chemotherapy and steroids can raise the risk for osteoporosis.

Rarely the condition can surface in children and teenagers, called juvenile osteoporosis. Sometimes a rare but severe variety can occur following childbirth, called pregnancy and lactation-associated osteoporosis (PLO).

Symptoms of Osteoporosis

Osteoporosis is symptomless initially, and individuals may learn about it only after a fracture. Sometimes, receding gums, diminished grip hold, and brittle nails have been found to precede the more eventful fractures.

A positive family history should alert you to the possibility of developing osteoporosis with age and menopause.

Fractures can occur anywhere, but the most typical locations are the following:

- Hip bones
- Vertebra
- Wrist bones
- Ribs

Symptoms of having a fracture are the following:

- Back pain
- Loss of height
- Loss of posture includes developing a stoop or a hunched back.

Osteoporosis Facts

The primary risk factor for osteoporosis is aging. About 1/10th of women above 60 and 2/5th above 80 have osteoporosis (Villiers & Goldstein, 2022).

- One in three women over 50 has an increased chance of osteoporotic fracture worldwide.
- Post-menopausal women are more affected by the condition than men of similar age. Loss of protective effects of hormones like estrogen is held responsible.
- The ratio of women to men osteoporotic fractures is 1.6; thus, 80% of forearm fractures and 70% of hip bone fractures occur in women.
- A previous fracture is associated with an 86% increased rate of subsequent fractures.
- Fragility fractures, especially hip fractures, are among the leading causes of morbidity.

Summary

- Osteoporosis is a bone condition with reduced bone density and bone mass.
- Bones become fragile and prone to fractures.
- Osteoporosis is more common in postmenopausal women.
- A family history of osteoporosis or hip fractures increases the risk of developing the condition.
- Osteoporotic fractures are the leading cause of morbidity.

The next chapter is on the prevention and management of osteoporosis.

Chapter Two

Osteoporosis Diagnosis

"Build better bones"

-2023 World Osteoporosis Day campaign slogan

Osteoporosis is a chronic illness that can lead to spontaneous bone fractures, even from minor incidents. The disease progresses silently, and fractures may be the first sign of its presence. It has considerable morbidity due to nagging pain, deformity, disability, and associated depression. To manage this damaging condition, you may undergo routine screening tests. These tests can determine your susceptibility to the disease and guide you on precautions to prevent it. Screening tests can also detect osteoporosis in its early stages when it may not yet be causing symptoms.

Screening For Osteoporosis

According to the U.S. Preventive Services Task Force, women in the following groups must routinely screen for osteoporosis. The Task Force did not recommend routine screening for men due to a lack of evidence for its benefit.

- Women who are more than 65 years of age.
- Women of any age with risk factors for osteoporosis.

You can assess your risk factors by answering the following questionnaire. These factors increase the chances of osteoporosis. They do not mean that you have the condition yet, but you must take precautions and undergo further tests for confirmation.

- Are you more than 60 years?
- Did you break your bones anytime after 50?

- What is your BMI? The body mass index or BMI is a measurement of body fat. To determine it, you have to divide your body weight by the square of height in meters. You can also use online calculators. A BMI less than 19 kg/m2 predicts weak bones. Being underweight can weaken the bones. You may also have lower estrogen levels than women with normal BMI.
- Did you lose height over the years? A loss of 4 cm is predictive of silent vertebral fractures.
- Did any of your parents have osteoporosis or a hip fracture? Parental history of osteoporosis or hip fracture increases your risk of osteoporosis.
- Are you a heavy drinker or smoker?
- Do you take medications like steroids, SSRIs, PPIs, or cancer medications?
- Do you have medical illnesses like thyroid disorders, inflammatory bowel disorders, chronic kidney failure, or rheumatoid arthritis? They can be associated with osteoporosis.

During a physical examination, your doctor will check your height, weight, posture, balance, and gait. They will also test your muscle strength using simple methods like your ability to stand from a seated posture without aid.

Fracture Risk Assessment Tool (FRAX) is an online tool that estimates a 10-year possibility of having a fracture after minor trauma. You may use it to learn your risk for fracture. You may have a doctor's consultation in case of a positive FRAX result. FRAX is useless if you already have a suspected fracture or are on medication for improving bone health.

Tests for Osteoporosis

There are no specific tests for osteoporosis. A bone mineral density (BMD) test measures bone mass and strength. Doctors typically test the hip bones and spine to see BMD. Its purpose is as follows:

- Diagnosis of osteoporosis

- Screening for prevention of osteoporosis. A reduced BMD is suspicious.
- Predictive of future fractures.
- Monitoring treatment usefulness.

The most common method for measuring BMD is dual-energy X-ray absorptiometry or DXA scan. Avoid calcium tablets one day before the test to prevent the likelihood of interference with scan results.

DXA scan is swift and painless. It does not require any procedure. It generates low levels of X-ray, which is not harmful to the body tissues. You lie on an insulated table as the scanner tests the specific body parts.

Sometimes a portable peripheral DXA is used to check the wrist and heel bone density quickly. Although it is a helpful screening test, peripheral DXA cannot predict fracture risks or monitor the effects of therapy on bone density. Individuals with spinal or hip deformities may find lying on the examination table difficult. A Portable scan is a valid option for them.

Bone density in forearms can be less than in hips in individuals with hyperfunctioning thyroid and parathyroid glands. Doctors may suggest forearm bone density measurements for them.

Doctors compare The BMD results against the average bone density of young and healthy individuals and individuals corresponding to your age, gender, and ethnicity. Doctors can diagnose osteoporosis if your value is less than the standard value.

Other tests for osteoporosis include a quantitative ultrasound or QUS of the heel. The test measures bone mineral density and predicts hip, back, or wrist fractures. The radiation-free test is rapid and easy to perform.

Blood or urine tests can detect other medical conditions associated with osteoporosis. Additionally, serum calcium levels, vitamin D levels, and bone-specific alkaline phosphatase levels can be recommended to check the levels of overall bone formation.

Reasons for Repeating DXA

- Your initial bone scan shows a T-score of -2.00 to -2.49 at any location.
- For women 65 years of age and older with a T-score of -1.50 to -1.99 at any location during the initial screening, repeating the scan every 3 -5 years is recommended, even without risk factors for notable bone loss.
- For women 65 years of age and older with average or slightly lower bone mass and a T-score between -1.01 to -1.49 and without risk factors for significant bone loss, a follow-up DXA in 10 to 15 years is recommended.
- You are on medications that reduce bone mass.
- You have medical conditions adversely affecting bone density.
- You have osteoporosis and are on medications.

In the last three instances, doctors can recommend repeating bone scans every two years to assess bone health, development of the illness, or therapy progress (Finkelstein, 2023). Preferably do the follow-up DXA in the same place as before to maintain parity between findings.

Bone Density

Bone density measures bone mass and strength. The "T" or "Z" scores represent the results of a bone density test. T-scores are numbers that compare your bone density to that of an average young individual with healthy bones. Z-scores are also numbers, but they show how your bone health is in comparison to an average individual of *your age*. The T score is more vital than the Z score.

T score numbers are negative or minus; the lower the score, the more the risk of fractures.

Normal Bone Density

Individuals having normal bone density show a T- score between +1 and -1. If your T-score falls in this range and you are above 50, you must take precautions to prevent bone loss by caring for your habits and lifestyle.

Osteopenia

Osteopenia is a condition of low bone mass. The bone density is less than average but is not yet in the osteoporotic range. The T-score typically falls between -1.1 and -2.4. If you are osteopenic, you have an increased chance of osteoporosis. The hazard is higher in the presence of other risk factors. The therapy, in this instance, is also directed toward preventing osteoporosis, but it is more emphatic than when the T-score results are normal. Doctors may prescribe medications for you, depending on the situation.

Osteoporosis

Your T-score is -2.5 or less. Since this is a negative score, a value of -3.0 would signify poorer scores than -2.5. Higher scores will veer toward -1.0. The therapy, in this case, is medications and lifestyle changes like diet, supplementation, and weight-bearing exercises.

A history of a bone fracture following minor trauma establishes an osteoporosis diagnosis, notwithstanding your bone density T-score. The doctors can prescribe specific medications to treat the condition, besides advising lifestyle changes and exercise.

Summary

- Women over 65 years of age and women of any age with risk factors for osteoporosis must be screened for the condition.

- A BMI less than 19 kg/m2 predicts weak bones.
- A loss of 4 cm is predictive of silent vertebral fractures.
- DXA scan is for osteoporosis diagnosis and monitoring treatment benefits.
- The T-score in osteopenia falls between -1.1 and -2.4. The aim of therapy is the prevention of osteoporosis.
- The T-score is -2.5 or less in osteoporosis. The aim of therapy is the treatment of the condition and fracture prevention.

In the next chapter, we will discuss in some detail about prevention and management of osteopenia and osteoporosis.

Chapter Three
Osteoporosis Management & Prevention

"Osteoporosis is treatable, if not preventable."

-Stuart J. Fischer, MD.

Fischer emphasized that irrespective of age; you must care for your bone health and take every step to protect and improve it.

Prevention of osteoporosis

The primary aim of any intervention for any condition, including osteoporosis, is disease prevention. It means you stop the disease even before it takes root in your body. Considering that it is a silently progressive disease, the natural question is how to prevent it. The other factor to ponder is some amount of bone loss is natural with age. In this regard, the primary prevention for osteoporosis would be to slow down the process of bone loss. Is it possible?

The first step in prevention is awareness. Knowing what osteoporosis is, its risk factors and your risks for having it can go a long way in taking steps to reduce the rate of progression of bone loss with age. The second step is action. We adopt measures to stall bone loss or reduce the rate of loss that is natural with age. The preventative measures can be exercises to improve posture, muscle strength, and balance.

Positive lifestyle changes like smoking cessation, drinking, adequate sleep, and proper diet can rebuild bone strength. The third step is the maintenance of activities and habits that foster bone health.

In this chapter, we will discuss each of these methods in detail.

Exercise

The human body is meant for exercising. Exercise is crucial to our body, including the mind and spirit. We know it reduces stress, removes boredom, and makes us feel accomplished, healthy, safe, and cared for. Such positive vibes go a long way in establishing other more fundamental benefits of exercise on cardiovascular, bone, and neurological health.

Whether or not you are susceptible to osteoporosis, exercise is your best ally to maintain bone health. The stress of exercise is good for maintaining the normal cycle of bone breaking down and formation.

But any exercise is not equally beneficial for preventing osteoporosis. The exercise tailor-made for the condition has to be weight-bearing, which improves bone density. It includes exercises we do, standing on our feet, and the muscles and bones working against gravity. The muscles and tendons put traction on the bones. The bones make more bone tissues in the face of this challenge. Thus, osteopenia and osteoporosis risks are reduced.

Accordingly, *gymnastics* and *weightlifting* exercises have the most significant impact on improving bone density. *Yoga* and also *chair yoga* incorporate both these components. Other components like rate and frequency of strain during exercises like jumping or running are challenging to sustain continuously without injuring our bones, tendons, and ligaments and are best avoided.

Our bone health is like a bank. The more you earn and deposit in your youth, the better you stay after retirement. An exercise regimen is most fruitful when started early, as the peak bone density is reached by age 30. However, there is no alternative to routine exercise at any age to keep your bones, body, and mind fresh and energetic.

Weight-Bearing Exercise

Weight-bearing exercise is any exercise that exerts a force on a bone. You use your body weight against gravity. The load of gravity on your bones stimulates bone cells to replace weak areas. Thus, working against gravity makes our bones strong. Astronauts working in zero gravity of outer space or in reduced gravity in spaceships can lose bone. We also lose bones when we avoid weight-bearing exercise and largely live sedentary lives. Regular weight-bearing activities in youth can prevent bone loss and strengthen bones. The muscles are strengthened, and posture is well-maintained.

Some examples of weight-bearing exercises are as follows:

- Walking on level ground or a treadmill
- Walking in place, holding the back of a chair for balance
- Sit-to-stand exercises. Start from a raised seat and progress to a lower chair as your bones strengthen.
- Stand against a wall and bend your knees, sliding down. Hold the position for 10 seconds, and repeat a few times. Hold the back of a chair for support.
- Weight-lifting lying down to support your back
- Strength training like push-ups, squats, lunges, etc.
- Climbing stairs
- Aerobics or dancing like Zumba
- Gymnastics
- Racquet sports
- Last but not least, yoga and Tai Chi. They improve balance and stability.

Mixed-up Exercise

Mixed-up movements challenge your body to move in different directions, forward, sideways, and backward. You perform skips, hops, and jumps or do any activity that teases your brain and body. Do these activities on level grounds in comfortable and secure environments. Doing them can reduce bone loss and maintain position sense and balance.

Weight Lifting

Weight lifting on its own accord is not sufficient for improving bone density. However, it can help you manage your body weight and enhance your metabolism. As a bone-strengthening activity, it is better than non-impact training like swimming. Research shows that only lower-body strength training exercises are less helpful than combined upper and lower-body strength training exercises.

In post-menopausal women, using vibration platforms for five minutes thrice a week can improve bone density in the spine by 2% compared to those who do not use them (Thompson, 2014).

Lifestyle changes

Stop Smoking: Smoking excessively increases osteoporosis in various ways. Bone-forming cells cannot work efficiently, and estrogen's protective action on bone tissues is negatively affected. It also amplifies the risks of injuries and fracture healing. Smoking reduces appetite and body weight, which can harm bone health.

Restrict alcohol: The recommended amount of alcohol is 1 or less drink daily for women and 2 or less for men. Excessive drinking affects appetite, nutrition, and body coordination. Alcohol interferes with the absorption of calcium and vitamin D. Estrogen action and action of bone-forming cells are reduced. Alcohol can cause neurological problems, which in turn affects gait and posture.

Take care of sensory organs: Regular checking of vision and hearing is essential in postmenopausal women. Visual problems increase falls and injuries. Visual acuity decreases with age, cataract formation, and other eye problems can occur.

Sensory-neural deafness commonly occurs with aging. Hearing loss affects posture and balance.

Prevent falls: Chances of losing balance and falls increase with aging. Unfamiliar environments increase the risks of falls.

The home environment must have sufficient safety and security features like proper lighting and ventilation. Change rugs and carpets with holes or loose ends and unsafe furniture and fittings. Floors and shower areas must be non-slip. Handrails and walking sticks should be used whenever necessary. Yoga and Tai chi improve balance and prevent falls.

Encourage hobbies: It is always better to stay engaged in doing something you love. Your jobs sustained you, but retirement is for doing things you previously had no time for. Some hobbies like gardening and nature walking combine exercise with mindful meditation. Volunteering for different organizations in your community can be bonding and uplifting.

Healthy diet: Eat three meals and two snacks, and drink plenty of water.

Sleep: Adequate rest and sleep for 7 - 8 hours at night are essential to maintain your overall health. Sleep improves focus and motivation for routine activities.

Diet

Calcium and vitamin D improve bone health. Foods rich in calcium include dairy products, tofu, nuts and seeds, dark leafy vegetables, and cruciferous veggies like cabbage, bok choy, and cauliflower. Postmenopausal women need 1200 mg of calcium daily (How can I get enough calcium, 2013). A diet plan containing 1000 mg of calcium per day would look like this:

- One pot of yogurt (200 g)
- One serving of muesli (50 g) with milk (100 ml)

- One slice of rye bread or whole-grain bread
- One slice (30gm) of gouda, edam or emmental cheese
- One serving (160 gm) of green cabbage
- One glass (200 ml) of mineral water.

vitamin D is produced by exposing our skin to sunlight. From March to the end of September, sunlight exposure directly on your skin between 10 am to 4 pm for 10 - 20 minutes daily is sufficient to produce vitamin D. Fatty fish and, to some extent, beef liver and cheese are food sources of vitamin D. Supplements of vitamin D are available as OTC products and use them in the winter months, or if exposure to the sun is not possible.

Adequate protein requirements for healthy postmenopausal women is 1.1g/kg body weight/day (Gregorio, 2014). Foods rich in best quality proteins include eggs, fish, and lean meat. Plant protein sources are tofu, beans, nuts and seeds, yogurt, and legumes.

Stress Management

Stress impacts poorly on our immune systems, making us vulnerable to infections and other health problems. It reduces the action of hormones, and that can affect bone health. Stress management is an active process. Some ways of stress therapy include meditation, yoga, spending time in nature, engaging in some hobbies, and learning new things. Bond socially and spend some time away from electronic technologies. As the best medicine, laughter can be embraced to lighten moods.

Treatment of Osteoporosis

Your doctors can prescribe medications for osteoporosis. Most of these drugs cannot replace the bones you have lost. But they are effective in preventing fractures and disability. Medications reduce the rate of bone loss by diminishing the action of the bone-breaking osteoclasts. Those who need medications include the following individuals:

- Postmenopausal women and men over 50 years with one or more of the following:
- Fracture spine
- Fracture hip
- T score of the hip or spine determined by a DXA scan shows a value of -2.5 or worse, indicating osteoporosis.
- T score of -1 to -2.5 in the hip or spine, signifying osteopenia and increased fracture risk.

The following categories of medications are available for osteoporosis:

- **Bisphosphonates** drugs like alendronate, risedronate, ibandronate, and zoledronic acid slow bone resorption or bone loss and improve bone health.
- **Selective estrogen receptor modulators (SERMs)** are estrogen derivatives that build bone strength. Synthetic estrogens like raloxifene with estrogen-like action build new bone tissues and are used in some postmenopausal women.
- **Calcitonin** is a natural hormone that controls the body's calcium levels. Doctors can prescribe it for painful broken bones in the spine. It is used as a nasal spray.
- **Denosumab** is a monoclonal antibody that prevents bone loss, reducing the risk of fractures. It only targets specific cells in the body.
- **Anabolic agents** like Teriparatide and abaloparatide are synthetic forms of the natural human parathyroid hormone or PTH. They stimulate the body to build new bones. You can self-inject them under the skin of the thigh or lower stomach once daily for up to 2 years. Anabolic drugs are available in prefilled dosing pens.
- **Estrogen replacement therapy** was the only FDA-approved treatment for *preventing* osteoporosis. Although there are concerns for increased chances of breast cancer, stroke, heart attacks, blood clots, and uterine cancer, estrogen

replacement therapy is used even now to preserve bone mass and prevent fractures in postmenopausal women only.

Summary

- Lifestyle changes like smoking cessation, drinking, adequate sleep, and proper diet can rebuild bone strength.
- Meditation and yoga can reduce stress and hormonal imbalance, affecting bone health.
- Weight-bearing exercises build bone density and strength.
- Some weight-bearing exercises include walking, running, aerobics, and yoga.
- Yoga improves body posture and balance.

The next chapter is on the first set of weight-bearing chair yoga exercises, which can improve bone health.

Chapter Four

Weight-Bearing Chair Yoga Exercises

"Yoga allows us to reach the goal of life that is to live worthy."

-Yoga guru, B.K.S. Iyengar

The best physical activities to build bone density and strength are weight-bearing exercises. However, some of them, like jumping, running, and jogging, can damage weakened bones. Activities that require rapid changes in body posture or direction, like aerobics or movements that involve deep extension, flexion, and twisting of the spine, can be risky and can cause injuries or falls.

A Harvard University scientific analysis reported that yoga, especially Hatha yoga, through chair-based movements, improved body strength. The analysis scrutinized 33 studies, participated by more than 2000 volunteers above age 65. Yoga enabled better walking speed and the ability to rise from a chair (Lowenthal et al., 2023). Given that frailty is one of the significant issues with advancing age, yoga and chair yoga maintain body activity, and improve strength and flexibility.

Yoga is inexpensive and accessible. It does not need any preparation except a few warm-up stretches. You do not require any tools or gadgets except a hardback chair without hand rests for these yoga activities.

Yoga elevates our mood. This is because yoga's moves reflect the motion we see in nature. These rhythmic body movements attuned to your breath and body increase awareness of the immediate environment. Kinesthetic awareness is understanding our joints and body's position with all our senses. We develop an intuitive as well as factual knowledge of our surroundings and their relationship with the body, which gives us confidence. Confidence goes a long way in building health, encompassing the body, mind, and spirit.

Essentially, yoga mimics the movements of an infant, exploring the world through curious actions and understanding them concerning their body.

What is the role of gentle 10-minute chair yoga exercises in building bone strength? Just doing 10 minutes of yoga a day can improve bone density. Several studies show better T-scores on DXA scans after consistent yoga practice for 10 -12 minutes daily (Fisherman, 2009).

Before going into the postures themselves, mentioning a few notes of caution would be appropriate.

- If you have osteoporosis, ask your doctor about your best exercise options.
- Avoid asanas with extreme forward or backward bends or exercises that curve the spine, like back crunches with your chin and neck extended, touching your toes from a standing position, or pulling the knees to your chest.

Beginner Level

The following 8 yoga asanas are suitable for the beginners.

Easy Pose

Warm-Up & Grounding

Start your 10-minute yoga routine with the easy pose or sukhasana.

Method

You need a chair with a wide seat for this pose. Alternatively, you can sit on a low, wide bench.

- Sit on the chair with your legs in front of you.

- Fold your legs to sit cross-legged; each foot should be under the opposite knee.
- Sit tall in this pose, your eyes closed, and breathe deeply.

Benefits

- Strengthening of core abdominal muscle and back muscles.
- Stretching of thighs and inner groin.
- Calming and deeply relaxing.

Contraindication

- Tightness of hips, weakness of the knees, and acute low back pain.
- Injuries or surgery of knee or hip.

Variation

Sukhasana with side bend

Add strength to the pose by raising your hand left hand overhead.

- Your right hand should be on the left knee.
- Follow your left hand as you exhale and take your arm as much as possible over your head toward the right.
- Repeat on the other side.

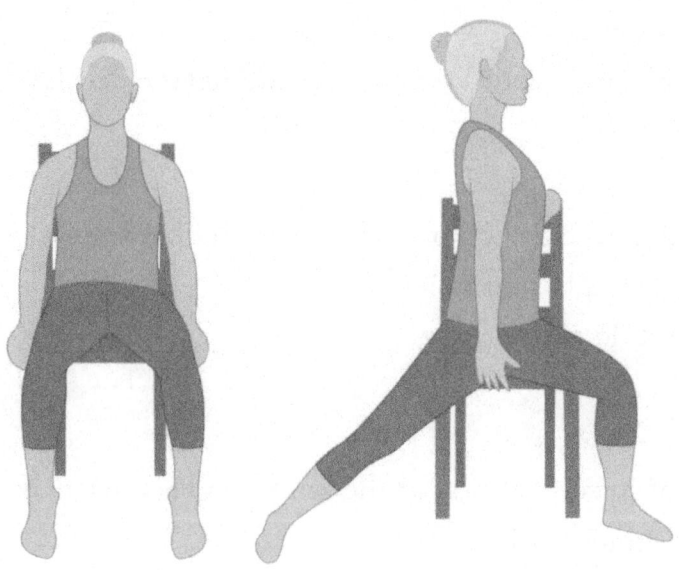

Chair Tiger pose

Strengthening & Balance

The tiger pose is called Vyagrasana in Sanskrit. The pose is great for core strengthening, balance, and stretching. Do the pose slowly, gradually adapting to it.

Method

- Sit sideways in a chair.
- Engage the core muscles by tightening the abdominals.
- Place both hands on your knees for support.
- Inhale and slowly arch your back, opening up your chest and lifting the chin as in the cow pose. Simultaneously, extend your outward leg backward as far as possible.
- Hold the position for 3 - 5 breaths.

- As you exhale, fold forward, rounding your back like a cat pose. Simultaneously, fold the outside leg toward your nose as far as possible.
- Hold the position for 3 - 5 breaths.
- Release.
- Repeat on the other side.

Benefits

- Core strengthening
- Stretches the abdominals.
- Opens the chest.

Contraindication

- Recent abdominal surgery.
- Injuries of the neck, shoulder, back, hips, or abdomen.

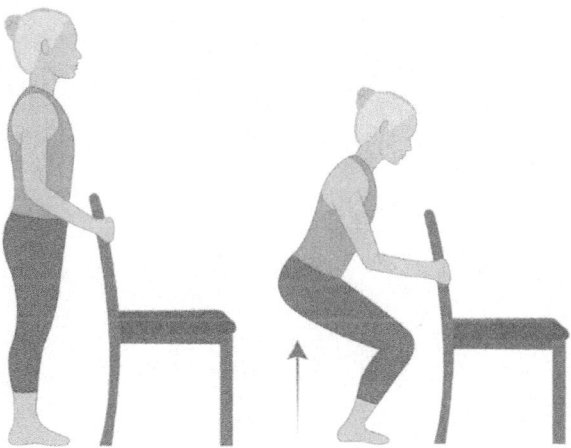

Mountain Pose Chair to Chair Flow

Core Strengthening

Tadasana to Utkatasana yoga is part of Vinyasa yoga. You will do the asana standing behind a chair.

Method

- Stand tall behind a chair, holding its back. Keep your feet hip-width apart.
- Open your chest and roll back your shoulders.
- Engage your core by tightening your belly button, and gradually bend your body at the hips, holding the chair all the while.
- Your body now resembles a chair.
- Hold the posture for 5 - 8 breath counts and release.

Benefits

- Core strengthening and grounding.

Contraindication

- Injuries of back and hips.
- Dizziness.

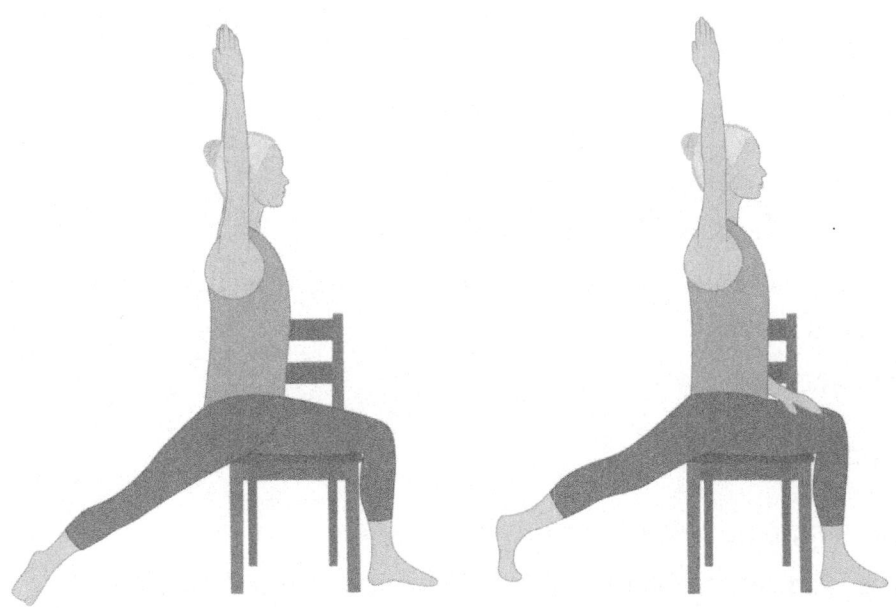

Chair Warrior I

Balancing & Strengthening

This pose is called virabhadrasana in Sanskrit. You become more aware of your body's position with the movements. This awareness restores your body's alignment and balance. You gain confidence and strength.

Method

- Sit tall, facing forward, on a chair without touching its back. Your arms are down by your sides, forming a low and wide angle, which is more straightforward for those who find it difficult to straddle the chair.
- Or, straddle the seat with one leg across the chair, your body facing forward.
- Inhale deeply, and gradually raise your arms straight above your head.
- Hold the posture for 3 - 5 breaths.
- Lower your arms to your sides.

- Repeat the asana on the opposite side if you do this pose with one leg across the chair.

Benefit

- Improves balance and position sense.
- Stretches thigh, hips, chest, and back muscles.
- The asana opens up the hip for those who can sit astride the chair. It can relieve sciatica pain.
- It energizes the body.

Contraindication

- Injuries to hip, knees, back, and shoulder.
- If there is a neck problem, hold the neck in a neutral position.
- If there is a shoulder problem, bring your arms to your sides parallel to the ground instead of lifting them.

Chair Warrior II

Balancing & Strengthening

This asana is called virbhadrasana II in Sanskrit.

Method

- Sit astride the edge of a chair, facing the right side and balancing yourself well.
- Inhale, raising your arms above your head.
- As you exhale, open your arms, your right hand facing you and carrying your left hand back.
- Reposition your trunk by drawing the left hip backward, and tilting a little to the left, so that your trunk is aligned with the chair's front.
- Hold the asana for 3 breaths.
- Release and relax.

- Do the movements on the other side.

Benefit

- Strengthening of legs and arms.
- Opens up the chest and shoulders.
- Toning for the abdomen.

Just as our body needs toning and strengthening, our facial muscles, too, require a workout. These last two chair yoga exercises maintain the vitality of our faces.

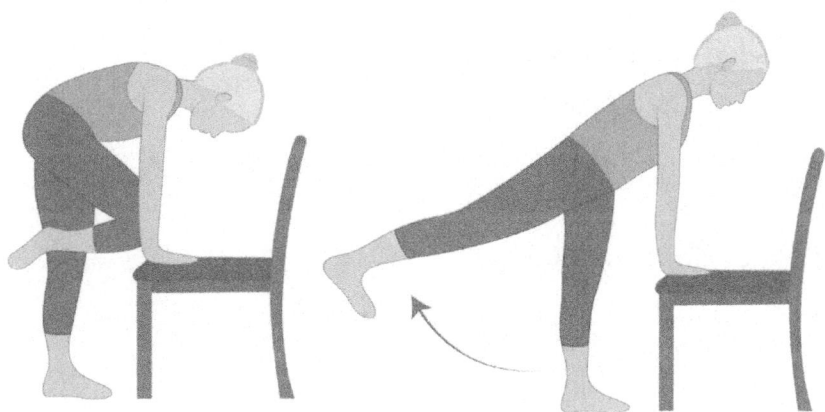

Table Top

Balance & Strengthening

The table top pose, or Varmanasana is done standing. You can use a chair to do the pose.

Method

- Stand tall in the mountain pose facing a stable chair.
- Bend down, resting the palms of both hands on the seat of the chair.
- Inhale and gently lift the left leg from the floor. Your ight leg rests on the ground.
- Extend it backwards, toes pointing down.
- Tighten the belly button.
- Hold the pose for 5 - 10 breaths.
- Release and repeat on the other side.

Benefit

- Strengthens leg and core muscles.
- Helps in balance and posture.

Contraindication

- Injury to knee, foot, and ankle.
- Vertigo.

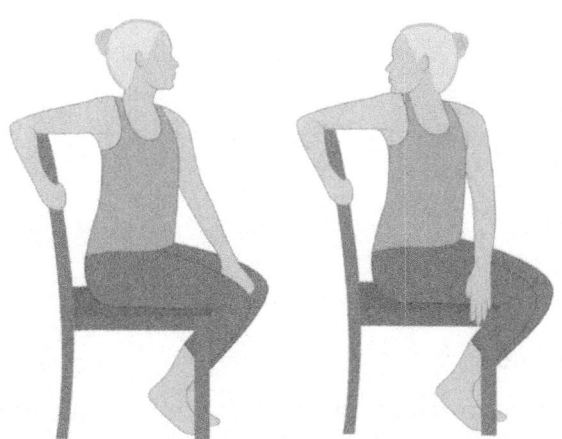

Seated Twist

Back Strengthening & Lengthening

This asana is called ardha matsyandresana in Sanskrit. It strengthens, stretches, and lengthens the muscles of the spine.

Method

- Sit sideways, facing left on the chair without touching its back.
- Inhale and lengthen your spine.
- As you exhale, slowly twist your body to the left side, your face toward the left. Hold to the back of the chair for support.
- Inhale, lengthen your spine and twist to the left on exhalation.
- Repeat the movement 3 - 5 times.
- Turn to your right and carry out the asana on this side 3 - 5 times.

Benefit

- Lengthening of the spine.
- Improves flexibility.
- Improves back pain.

Contraindication

- Obesity.
- Knee problems.
- Injuries in the tailbone.
- Individuals unable to coordinate body movement with breathwork.

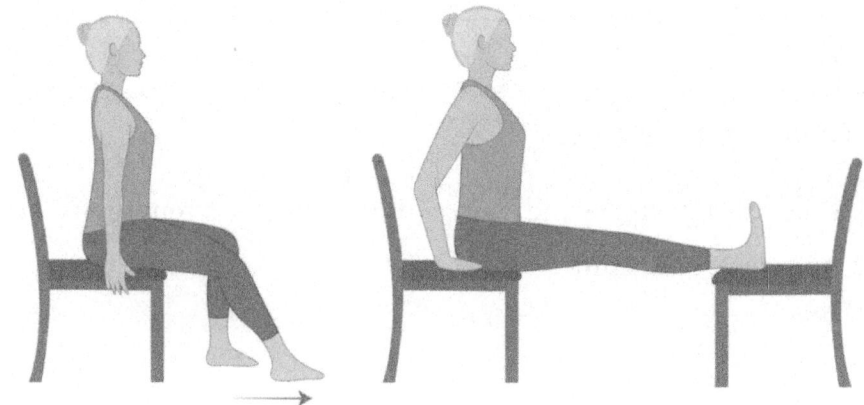

Staff Pose

Stability

Also called dandasana, staff pose needs a chair with armrests and a bench or a stool the same height as the chair's seat.

Method

- Place the bench or the stool in front of the chair.
- Sit tall on the chair and lift both legs on the stool or the bench, stretching your legs in front of you. Take the help of the armrests if needed.
- Shift your position to sit on your tailbone.
- Your thighs, knees, feet, and ankles should be held together.
- Your palms should be on the chair's side, fingers pointing forward.
- Lock your elbows.
- Lift your chest.
- Tighten the core and thigh muscles, tugging them toward your groin.
- Press down your thighs on the chair, and hold your head, neck, and hips in one straight line.
- Hold the posture for 5 - 8 breath counts.

Benefit

- Strengthens chest muscles.
- Tones core, back, and thigh muscles.
- Lengthens leg ligaments.

Contraindication

- Back, knee, or leg injury or surgery.

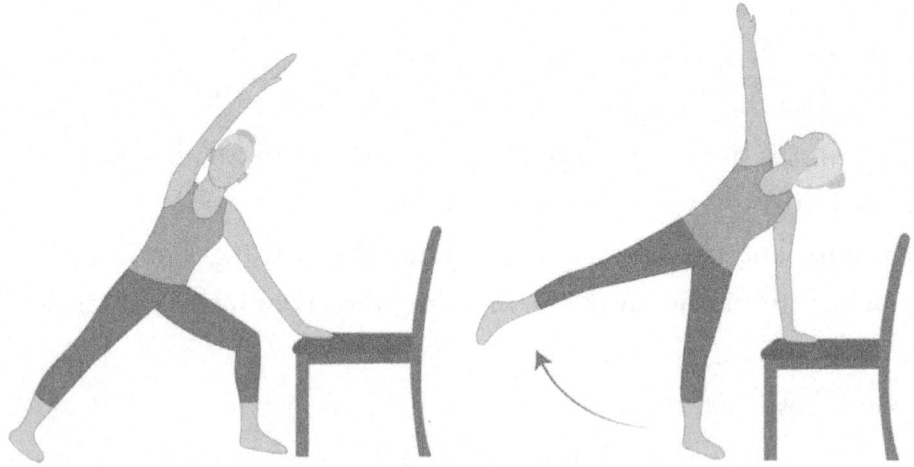

Intermediate Level

Half-Moon

Strengthening & Stability

Also called ardha-chandrasana, the half-moon pose is an intermediate-level yoga suitable for strengthening and lengthening the body.

Method

- Stand tall, facing a stable chair.
- Inhale, raise your arms on exhale, push your hips out, pull in your belly, and lower both arms on the chair's seat.
- Inhale, slowly take your right leg behind you, and slightly bend your left knee.
- Hold the position for 2 - 3 breaths. Align the right leg with the hip, the left leg with the ankle, and the shoulders with the forearms.
- Lift the right leg behind you, parallel to the floor, breathing slowly and deeply. Straighten the left leg.

- Lift the right arm from the chair, supporting your body with your left arm on the chair's seat.
- Slowly turn your body to look up toward the right arm.
- Hold the position for 5 - 8 breaths and turn round.
- Lower your right arm and return your right leg to its original position.
- Repeat with the other side.

Benefit

- Body strengthening and lengthening exercise.
- Restores balance.
- Addresses back pain.
- Opens up the chest and improves respiratory functions.

Contraindication

- Unsuitable for beginners.
- Injuries in the exercising body parts.

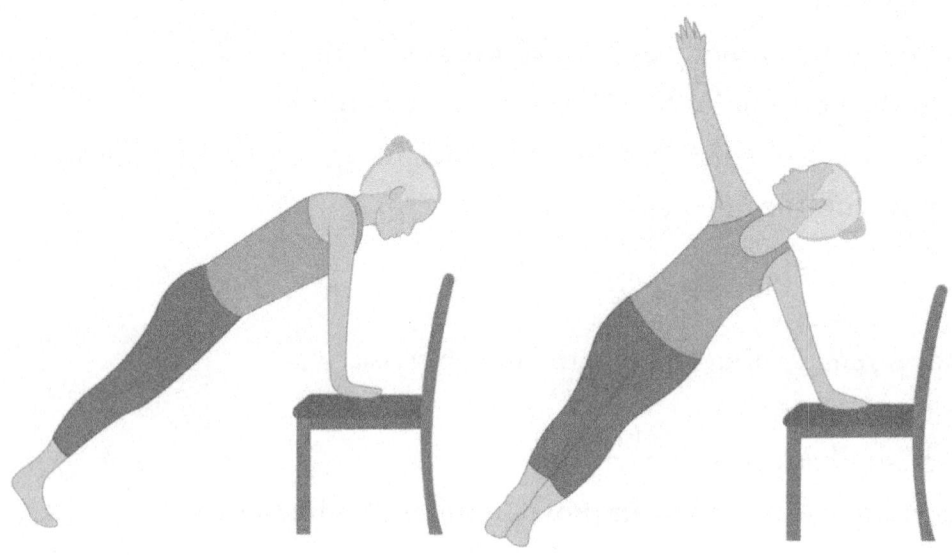

Side-Plank Pose

Strengthening

The Sanskrit name for this asana is vasisthasana, which is to hold your body sideways, one hand resting on a chair.

Method

- Take a stable chair to support the weight of upper body.
- Start the asana with the table top sequence, your palms must be on the chair's seat.
- Step backward, keeping your knees straight and feet planted on the ground. Feel the stretch on the calf muscles.
- Gradually turn on your right side, and raise your right arm toward the ceiling.
- Your body now forms an inclined line with the floor, supported by the left hand on the chair.

- Hold the pose for 5 - 8 breaths.
- Release and repeat on the other side.

Benefit

- Strengthening and lengthening for back and leg muscles.
- Awareness of balance.
- Energizing.

Contraindication

- Injury and recent surgery of the back, neck, and limbs.

Virasana

Strengthening

In Sanskrit, Virasana means warrior. The asana is good for strengthening and endurance.

Method

You will need a chair and a bolster for the chair Virasana.

- Sit in a chair, after placing a bolster behind the front legs of the chair.
- Bend your feet at the knees and thrust them under the chair, resting the front of the ankles on the bolster.
- Stretch your spine, your shoulders are above your hips.
- Raise your arms toward the ceiling, interlocking the fingers.
- Your chest is open and your chin is up.
- Breathe into the posture for 5 - 8 breaths before relaxing.

Benefit

- Strengthening of the spinal muscles.

- Relieves backache
- Reduces pain in the tailbone.

A variant of Virasana

With Chair as a Support

Method

- Sit on your knees on a mat behind a chair.
- Your feet should be behind you, the soles facing the ceiling.
- Hold the back of the chair to sit on your feet. The outer surfaces of the thighs should touch the inner aspects of the calf muscles.
- Gradually lower your hips to the floor between your feet. Your weight should be on the thighs.
- Lift up your chest, and sit tall. Hold the back of the chair for support.
- Hold the pose for 5 - 8 breaths and relax.

Parsva Virasana

Strengthening

Parsva Virasana means sidewise warrior pose. The asana improves the strength of the feet, improves digestion, and improves blood flow to the spine.

Method

- Sit in a chair, after placing a bolster behind the front legs of the chair.
- Bend your feet at the knees and thrust them under the chair, resting the front of the ankles on the bolster.
- Stretch your spine, your shoulders are above your hips.
- Exhale, placing the left hand on the outer side of the right thigh.
- Take your right hand toward the right hip reaching your back.

- Slowly turn toward the right, giving a beautiful twist to your spine. Tuck your shoulders back, and your neck should be relaxed.
- Hold the position for 5 - 8 breaths and relax.
- Repeat the posture on the other side.

Benefit

- Improves lower back pain.
- Strengthens arches of foot and spine.

Contraindication

- Migraine, vertigo, or headaches.
- Uncontrolled blood pressure.

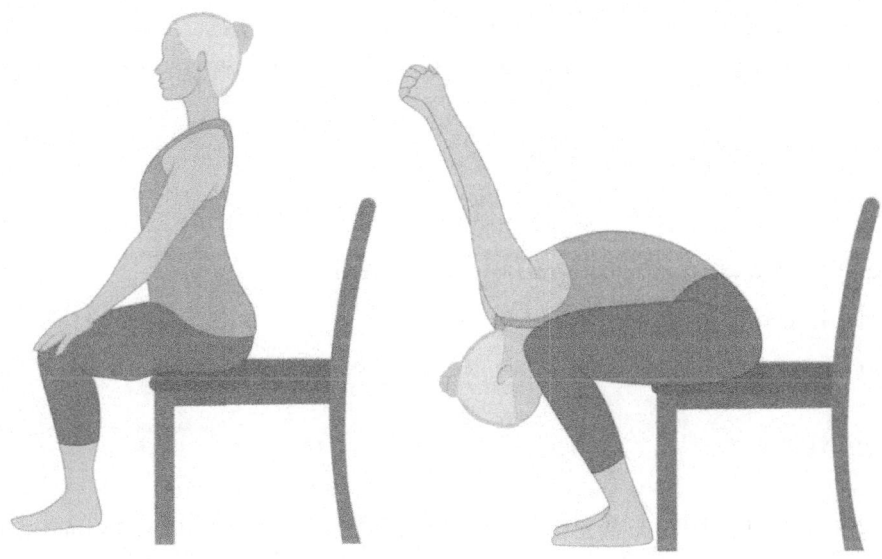

Volcano Pose

Strengthening

The volcano pose or urdha hastasana is a good posture to strengthen the core and improve stability.

Method

- Sit upright, in a seated mountain pose
- Keep your knees parallel to the ground over the ankles. There should be a small gap between them.
- Inhale deeply. Upon exhalation, roll your shoulders downward.
- Inhale again and this time, raise your hands toward the ceiling, joining the palms in *namaste* mudra.
- Lift your gaze to look up.
- Hold the position for 5 - 10 seconds.
- Release by bringing your neck to center, and then dropping the arms to your sides.

Benefit

- Strengthen the core, shoulders, and back muscles.
- Improve balance and flexibility.
- Improves breathing.

Contraindication

- Acute pain and trauma of the shoulder and neck joints and muscles.

Summary

- Use a stable chair without an armrest.
- The chair should rest firmly on the ground and be able to carry your weight.

- Begin yoga with a warm-up, and end with a cool-down.
- Introduce yourself to the asanas slowly without exerting yourself.
- Start with three to four asanas, and repeat each two to three times. Gradually increase the frequencies and repetitions.

The next chapter discusses a few more asanas suitable for bone strength and stability.

Chapter Five

Gentle Yoga for Osteoporosis

"Yoga teaches us to cure what need not be endured and endure what cannot be cured."

- B.K.S. Iyengar

Yoga is not a religious practice, although ancient Sanskrit-speaking people of India considered it a gateway to the body, mind, and spiritual connection. It is true that yoga opens up your body, energizes the mind, and uplifts your spirit. In that regard, yoga is a way of coordinated and holistic living.

Chair yoga, an adaptation of traditional yoga, is a brainchild of Lakshmi Voelker-Binder in 1982. Lakshmi was a certified yoga trainer. When one of her young students was diagnosed with arthritis which prevented her from participating in traditional yoga classes, Lakshmi engineered chair yoga postures for her to practice from the chair. Her mantra, "Get fit where you sit," has since inspired people worldwide.

Yoga means union, denoting the unification of the body, mind, and spirit. Practice these simple and gentle yoga methods to stay fit.

Gentle Yoga

Gentle chair yoga is a modified yoga technique. It is low-impact and easy to do.

Despite the name "Gentle Yoga," they are powerful enough to rejuvenate your overall well-being. At the same time, you are not left exhausted by the demand of physical exertion. It is suitable for the following individuals:

- Difficulties in bending.
- Difficulty in carrying weight.

- With a health condition that precludes heavy exercise.
- Poor joint conditions.
- Chronic low backaches.
- Difficulties in concentrating, balance, or flexibility.
- Sedentary lifestyle and deconditioned body, without endurance.

How does gentle yoga help in these conditions? It helps you in the following ways:

- Improvement in balance and posture.
- Strengthening of bones and muscles.
- Improvement in flexibility.
- Enhancement of endurance.
- Stress reduction.

You can do the exercises in the safety and comfort of your home. All you require is a stable chair without an armrest.

The following exercises will help you to relax, stretch, strengthen your bones and muscles, and improve your breathing. You can do them alone, unassisted, or with friends for company. Yoga is related to breathwork, which is stress-reducing. Deep exhalation induces the calmative parasympathetic nervous system and reduces blood pressure and levels of stress hormones like adrenaline.

Deep breathing also helps deliver oxygen to body tissues and remove wastes from the body.

Since yoga combines breath work with exercises; we call these asanas Thoughtful or Mindfulness exercises.

We will commence our yoga practice with Ujjayi, a mindfulness pranayama, which improves your focus on the present moment. Simultaneously, it will prepare you for subsequent asanas. Although a mindful warm-up, Ujjayi asana is dynamic and requires active participation. Your breath will sound like soft waves rolling toward the shore.

The rhythmic sound of your breath, similar to the movements of the gentle waves, will help you to settle into the yoga asanas.

Exercises You Avoid

Since osteoporosis makes your bones vulnerable to injuries, talk with your doctors before doing the asanas.

Avoid the following postures:

- Pulling your legs to your chest while lying down on your back.
- Headstands or *shirshasana*.
- The plow poses.
- Shoulder stands.
- The downward dog.
- Spinal twists.
- Jumping.
- Belly crunches.
- Postures that do not support your neck and spine or squeeze the spine.
- Avoid the boat pose if you have a weak neck and spine.
- Avoid exercises that place your body weight on the neck.
- If you feel *pain* while doing the poses, abandon them immediately.

Many people practicing yoga believe that concentration on breathing can quiet their minds and help them to be fully involved with their daily activities, including exercises. Hence, practice effortless breathing as you move your body for the rest of the asanas. Breathe in through your nose for 4 seconds, hold your breath for a while, and then exhale through the nose for another 4 seconds. Let your breathing be smooth and even.

Warm-Ups

Start gentle chair asanas with a few stretches to mold your body into the asanas.

Shoulders

- Sit tall in a chair.
- Bring the right arm across the body above your chest, supporting it at the elbow with your right elbow.
- Hold for 5 - 8 seconds.
- Release and repeat on the other side.
- Now roll your shoulders slowly, first in one direction and then in the other.

Chest

- Bring your arms to your front, the thumbs facing up.
- Move them toward each side, opening up the chest.
- Repeat 5 -10 times.

Bone Mobility

- Lift your right foot slightly off the ground.
- Make 10 circles first in one direction and then in another.
- Repeat with the other side.

Child Pose

Also called *Balasana*, the pose is profoundly grounding and calming. The word *Bala* means child in Sanskrit, and through your asana, you submit like a child to the higher force.

Method

- Sit tall, your feet at hip-width apart.
- Rest your hands on your thighs, palms facing down.
- Now, fold over and rest your forehead on your palms.
- Keep your body flat as far as possible.
- Breathe as you release all tension and relax your body.

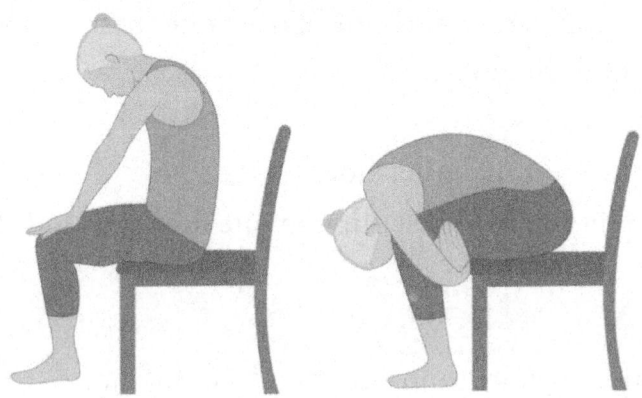

Variant

Child Pose

- You will need a low but long bench adequate for your body weight and height. Place a mat or rug on the bench for better support. You will need folded towels, cushions, and a chair for additional support as you sit on the bench.
- Sit on a bench with your legs folded behind you and your heels facing up. Support your body by holding the back of a chair.
- Now push back to place your hips on your heels. You can place a folded blanket under your knees.
- Slowly stretch your arms forward, folding and resting your head on the bench. Use a folded towel if your head doesn't reach the bench.

Benefit

- Calmative.

- Strengthens arms, shoulders, spine, and leg muscles.

Precaution

- Avoid doing the asana after meals.
- Low blood pressure.
- Vertigo.
- Neck problems.

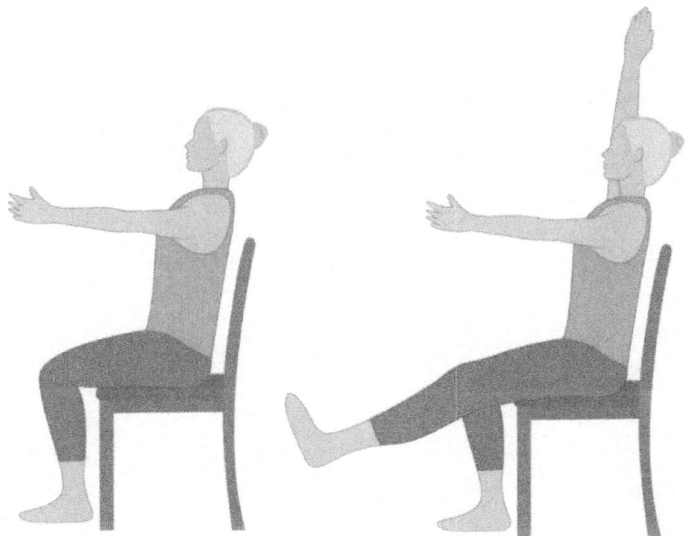

Dead Bug Core Exercises

This asana is a challenging pose that involves attention and coordiantion. The asana is done lying on a mat, but you can modify it for a chair exercise.

Method

- Sit tall toward the chair's front without touching its back. Your feet must be firm on the ground.
- Lift both legs to the air.

- Tighten your core and lift both arms upward.
- Exhale and bring the right leg down, simultaneously, lower your left hand.
- You should be sitting on your tailbone throughout the exercise.
- Hold the pose and in a flow of movements, raise the left arm, lowering the right one, and simultaneously, raise your right leg and lower the left one on the ground.

Benefit

- Imrpoves balance and coordination.
- Strengthens core muscles.

Precaution

- Back or neck problems.
- Hip surgery.

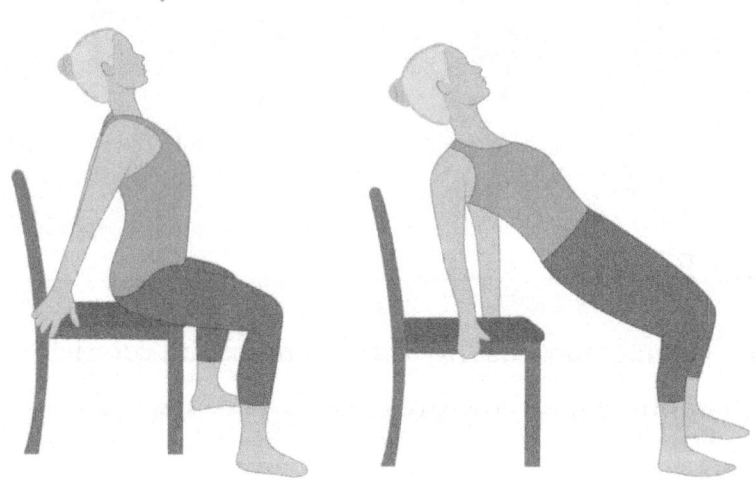

Camel Pose

Also called ustrasana in Sanskrit, you fold your body like a camel in this pose.

Method

- Sit tall on a chair; your back away from the chair's back.
- Keep your feet at hip-width apart on the ground.
- Position your hands behind you on the chair seat.
- Push your belly and chest forward.
- Roll back your shoulders and gaze at the ceiling.

Benefits

- Opens the chest.
- Strengthens core and stretches different muscle groups.
- Improves function of internal organs.

Precautions

- Avoid if you have neck, shoulder, and arm injuries.
- Dizziness and vertigo.
- Low blood pressure.

Variant

Camel Pose

Method

- Use a chair as support.
- Kneel on a mat and pull yourself to a sitting posture holding the back of a chair.

- Press your chest, belly, and hips forward and gently bend backward, trying to reach toward your heels and grab the shins with your hands.
- Roll back the shoulders and gaze upward.
- Hold the position for 5 - 8 seconds.

Boat Pose

Traditionally known as *paripurna navasana*, the boat pose helps in stability and core strength.

Method

- Sit sidewards on the chair.
- Squeeze the belly muscles and gently round your back. Support your body with your inner hand on the chair.
- Lift your chest, keep your spine straight, and lift one leg, slightly bent at the knee. Hold the back of the knee for support.
- Repeat on the other side.
- For an advanced pose, lift both legs straight into the air while holding onto the chair seat for support.

Benefit

- Strengthening of core, thigh, and spinal muscles.
- Improves stability.

Precautions

- Injuries of the back, hips, or arms.

Eagle Pose

Eagle pose, or garurasana, helps in stability and core strength.

Method

- Sit tall without touching the chair's back.
- Cross the right leg over the left and wrap them tightly.
- Bring your elbows forward to meet at your chest level.
- Cross your left wrist over the right to bring together the back of your hands. Your thumbs must be toward your nose.
- Squeeze the arms and the legs.
- Squeeze your core and lengthen your spine.
- Repeat by altering the position of the limbs.

Benefit

- Strengthens back and core muscles.
- Improves stability.
- Relieves stiffness of joints of the wrists and ankles.

Precaution

- Avoid the asana in wrist, ankle, leg, or arm injuries.

Crescent Lunge Position

It is the pose of the monkey god and is called *anjaneyasana* in Sanskrit.

Method

- Sit sideways on a chair.
- Stretch the outer leg backward, folding your toes under.
- Your front knee must be directly over your ankle.
- Raise arms toward the ceiling, holding them at shoulder-width.
- Lengthen your spine into the pose and tighten the core.
- Relax your shoulders
- Repeat on your other side.

Benefit

- Strengthens the legs and hips.
- Opens the chest.
- Improves flexibility.

Precautions

- Weak knees, ankles, shoulders, or hip joints.
- Vertigo.

Variant

Crescent Lunge Pose

Method

- Use a chair for balance.
- Stand with your feet at hip-width apart, holding the back of a chair.
- Place your right foot back comfortably and balance it on your toes, heels lifted.
- Bend your left leg, keeping your knee directly above the ankle.
- Holding the back of the chair with one hand, lift the other hand upward.
- Stretch your spine.
- Repeat on the other side.

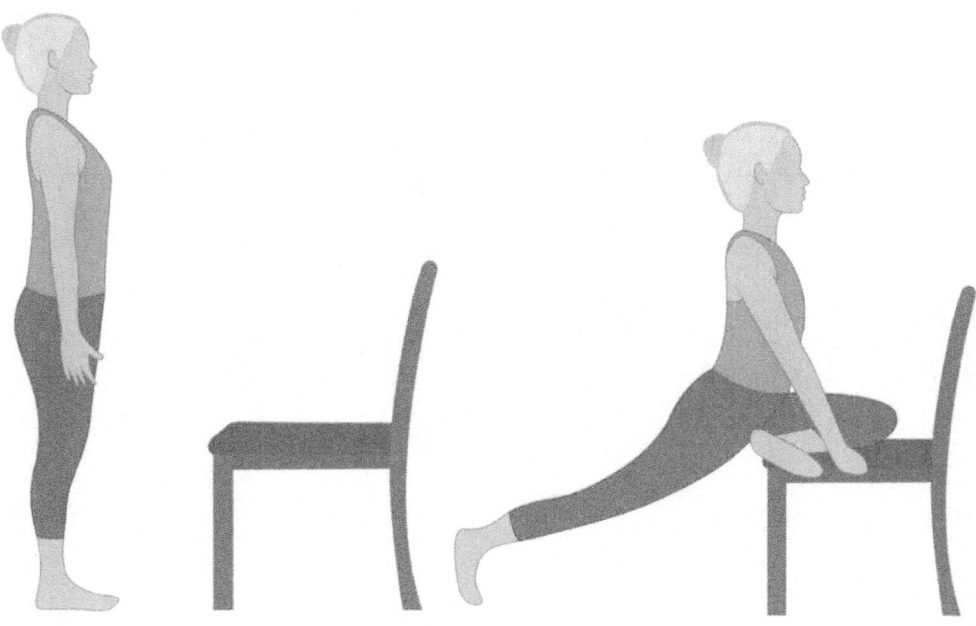

Half Pigeon Position

Traditionally called ardha-kapotasana, this pose is a Hatha Yoga practice with a mind=body connection.

Method

- Sit sideways on a chair.
- Lift the inside foot on the chair, folding it at the knee and holding the knee with both hands. Rest the inner hand on the chair's back in an advanced pose, and gently push the knee with the outer hand. Use blocks to raise the foot if necessary.
- Stretch the other leg back, straightening the knee as much as possible, and turn your toes under.
- Tighten the belly muscles, flatten the lower back, and sit tall.

- Repeat on the other side.

Benefit

- Strengthens hip and groin muscles.

Precaution

- Hip or knee injury.
- Rheumatoid Arthritis.

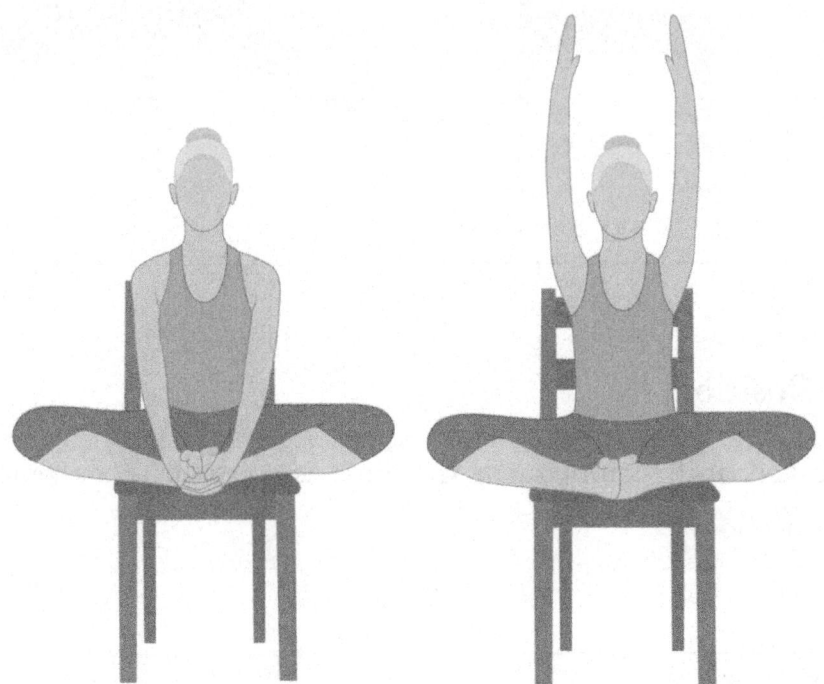

Cobbler Position

Its original Sanskrit name is Bhadrasana, and it opens your hips and strengthens the core.

Method

- Keep two chairs facing and touching each other.
- Sit toward the front of one chair.
- Place your feet on the second chair, folding them and touching one another at the heels. Your knees should be wide apart.
- Hold your ankles.
- Lengthen your trunk into the pose.

In an advanced pose, place your elbows on the inside of your thighs and fold forward at your hips. Keep the chin up and spine straight.

Benefit

- Strengthens the legs and hips.
- Opens the chest.
- Improves stability.

Precautions

- Weak knees, ankles, shoulders, or hip joints.
- Groin or knee injury.

Savasana

Cooling-Down

All yoga practices end with savasana, the deeply resting culminating pose. You use this asana to become aware of any tension or knots in your body, which must be released during this asana. use a chair to end your practice session with this restorative asana.

Method

- Sit on the chair; your eyes closed.
- Let your hands rest on your lap.

- Clear any tension from your mind.
- Allow your body to go limp.
- Breathe effortlessly as you relax in this resting pose.
- To release the posture, breathe deeply, curl your fingers and toes, and reach your hands toward the ceiling, giving a final stretch to your body.

Benefit

- Full body relaxation.
- Mindful awareness of the body.
- Assesses and releases muscle tension.
- Rejuvenates the body and the mind.

Conclusion

Osteoporosis and osteopenia are bone conditions that weaken your bones, increasing the risks of falls, accidents, and injuries. Moderation in lifestyles, foods rich in calcium, vitamin D supplements, and weight-bearing exercises can prevent it or reduce its impact on your lives.

However, if you already have the condition, you can check its progress by prompt medical care, nutrition, and exercise. Medications help prevent bone loss and pains due to fractures and injuries.

The 10-minute chair yoga methods mentioned in this book effectively prevent and manage osteoporosis. They are easy to do and practical without draining resources and time. Use them and enjoy doing them to stay strong and fit.

Printed in Great Britain
by Amazon